MW00625497

KILLER CARE

KILLER CARE

*How Medical Error Became
America's Third Largest Cause of Death,
and What Can Be Done About It*

JAMES B. LIEBER

OR Books

New York · London

© 2015 James B. Lieber

Published by OR Books, New York and London
Visit our website at www.orbooks.com

For all rights information: rights@orbooks.com

All rights reserved. No part of this book may be reproduced or transmitted in any
form or by any means, electronic or mechanical, including photocopy, recording,
or any information storage retrieval system, without permission in writing from
the publisher, except brief passages for review purposes.

First printing 2015

Cataloging-in-Publication data is available from the Library of Congress.
A catalog record for this book is available from the British Library.

ISBN 978-1-68219-010-4 paperback
ISBN 978-0-984295-09-8 e-book

Cover and text design by Bathcat Ltd.
Typeset by AarkMany Media, Chennai, India.
Printed by BookMobile in the United States and CPI Books Ltd in the United
Kingdom. The U.S. printed edition of this book comes on Forest Stewardship
Council–certified, 30% recycled paper. The printer, BookMobile, is 100%
wind-powered.

In Memoriam
Byrd R. Brown
(1930–2001)

CONTENTS

INTRODUCTION: Full Disclosure

L ike most Americans, I love and fear health care. With age, this fear increases. In fact, it increases reasonably. The old—I am 66—and the very young are more likely than other patients to suffer medical errors, including fatal ones.

I have a rare condition caused by a genetic mutation that puts me at risk of blood clots and stroke. A few years ago, when I was highly symptomatic, in great pain, and walking with difficulty, a doctor diagnosed this malady, which soon was confirmed by a blood test. I started taking a maintenance dose of oral chemotherapy, put aside my cane, and returned to a normal pain-free life with mobility.

A month before the accurate diagnosis, I had gone to an emergency room because of a gangrenous blackness on my foot and fear of a clot. The emergency physician wanted to admit me, and bring in a vascular surgeon to assess severing my toes. At this point, my family physician and a close friend appeared. With his backing I exercised the patient's essential right to say no, left the hospital, and saw a series of specialists, one of whom finally got it right.

Had my toes been amputated, I would have joined the ranks of those who have received wrong site, wrong limb, wrong organ, and other unnecessary surgeries known as "never events," because the medical profession admits that they never should have happened. Error specialists, and there are many, might say that I had a "near miss," something health care is just beginning to study and learn from following the example of the aviation industry.

I was fortunate, but others among my family and friends have not been so lucky. In her twenties, my future wife underwent an unneeded colonoscopy on a distressed and inflamed gut. The probe perforated her colon. This led to emergency surgery to save her life, a temporary colostomy, and subsequent surgeries to repair her intestine and remove the colostomy. She recovered fully, but went through a year of health-care hell. She endured an "overtreatment" error from an unnecessary procedure. As Sanjay Gupta, the neurosurgeon and chief medical correspondent for CNN, recently put it, "More treatment, more mistakes."

My father's later years were marred by a "hospital-acquired infection" (HAI) that he apparently contracted during a minor knee-draining procedure. My mother endured a "hand-off" error following surgery for a nonmalignant brain tumor. Because physicians failed to order anti-seizure medication, she convulsed and entered a coma for three weeks, from which she emerged a hemiplegic with limited speech. My close friend, the family practitioner who helped me avoid unnecessary foot surgery, saw his elderly mother enter but not leave the excellent teaching hospital where he serves on the staff. During routine cataract surgery, she suffered an anesthesia error, aspirated vomit, and died. My professional mentor, Byrd Brown, Pittsburgh's preeminent civil rights attorney, had a lung transplant at age 70. During the post-surgical hand-off, his attending physician ordered a necessary but highly toxic anti-rejection drug. A misplaced decimal point meant that my very sick colleague received ten times the intended dose. It killed him. A lethal prescription is regarded as a medication error.

Two of those situations led to medical malpractice claims that yielded settlements: one low and one moderate. I cannot say more because as in most civil tort claims, the eventual settlement and release documents contained clauses forever binding those involved to secrecy, which helps to resolve these grief-driven contests and soothes some of the suffering and loss with compensation, As controversial as they are common, such gag orders stop the public, patients, and health providers from learning as much as they might about medical accidents, and hopefully preventing them in the future.

Over four decades, I have pursued dual careers in law and writing. As an attorney I have concentrated on civil rights, employment, and business cases. Early on I was involved in a support role in a single medical malpractice case. A young couple sought genetic counseling at a world-renowned academic medical center in the South. Their first child had been stillborn and severely deformed. They wondered if they should attempt another pregnancy. They had excellent government insurance that covered this type of service because the husband was an active-duty soldier.

The geneticist who read the x-ray photomicrography of their chromosomes called a karyotype said that they were normal, healthy, and not at any greater risk than others. They conceived again, but this time the child was born alive, with major developmental defects that would require a lifetime of expensive care. It turned out that the geneticist misread their chromosomes. Prior to this he had analyzed only karyotypes of *drosophila* (fruit flies), not humans. Victims like these cannot be made whole in court and only rarely is their suffering fairly compensated, but this jury returned a large measure of damages to pay for the child's care. Again, I cannot say more because the case was resolved in such a way that the hospital decided not to appeal, and the family and its lawyers promised confidentiality. Nevertheless, everyone in and around this case learned a profound lesson about medical errors that has been vindicated by data: experience matters. Whether you are a patient in need of a lung transplant or merely seeking to have an x-ray read accurately, it makes total sense to pick a provider who has completed the task successfully many times before.

Of course, the vast majority of medical mistakes do not lead to lawsuits. However, the experiences just in my personal circle seem fairly typical. Medical errors touch many lives and frighten most of us. Almost everyone knows someone who has emerged from a hospital with an infection, or has read an obituary noting that a person died from "complications"—often a code word for medical error. A recent *Consumer Reports* poll found that 80 percent of hospital patients feared infections, and 65 percent were afraid of surgical error.

In 1999, the prestigious Institute of Medicine (IOM) of the National Academy of Sciences' book-length report *To Err Is Human: Building a Safer Health System* announced that 44,000 to 98,000 Americans died from medical errors annually, far exceeding the tolls from gun violence, suicide, AIDS, breast cancer, or automobile accidents. Commentators equated the carnage from health-care errors with the daily crash of a jumbo jet. This stark image produced some public attention, as did the IOM's call to halve these errors within five years, which was not to be. Now, *To Err is Human*'s statistics are regarded as conservative. Medical errors are a man-made epidemic, and it may be that only heart disease and cancer kill more of us.

In my career as an employment lawyer, I have represented many doctors, nurses, and other providers. This seems natural given that health care has swelled to over 22 percent of the economy. As a $2.7 trillion business, it impacts us all. Virtually everyone interfaces with the system as a patient, provider, payee, payor, family member, advocate, or friend. In terms of major medical interventions, the average American undergoes nine surgeries in a lifetime.

Doctors, nurses, and other medical staff must navigate an increasingly bureaucratic, technologically evolving, cost-driven, and chaotically managed environment where they win and lose positions in practices that can be bought, sold, or shunned by hospitals, which may themselves be folded into, spun out of, or shuttered by regional health-care systems. Funding for research to improve medical knowledge and safety, especially from the government, is entirely uncertain in an era of bean counting and fiscal cliffs.

One of my legal areas that has been an important window into error involves defending research doctors accused of scientific misconduct, which can result in their debarment from federal funds including millions of dollars in grants from the National Institutes of Health (NIH) supporting clinical studies and laboratories. These cases can lead to administrative trials before juries of scientists resulting in verdicts that can end brilliant careers in the fight against disease. Typically these clients have been the leaders of lengthy studies involving hundreds of patients and huge accumulations of information. Somehow, a data point has been lost or put in the wrong spot in a table or on a graph, or cannot be sourced. No patient has been harmed, but questions arise about the efficacy of potential or existing treatments. My cases have involved breast cancer, lead poisoning, and lupus, and included researchers who made mistakes rather than lied. At bottom, we often have understood that the errors emanated from communication flaws ("teamwork errors") in the lab or clinic that plague medicine but usually can be corrected. Also, sometimes personalities get in the way. Jealousies, ambitions, and bruised egos have led to cases, as on occasion have the habits and idiosyncrasies of very bright people who want to perform tasks their way rather than according to established standards and best practices.

As a writer, my assignments and storylines have involved assessing large industries. Some of these have included steel, agribusiness, finance, law enforcement, corrections, and health care, where in particular I have delved into fertility treatments and drug addiction. To my thinking, the best book on safety in modern industry is Ralph Nader's *Unsafe at Any Speed: The Designed-In Dangers of the American Automobile* (1965). In many ways, the mighty American car industry of the 1960s dominated by General Motors foreshadowed the health-care colossus of today. Our postwar car industry was the biggest in the world. It had no real foreign competition, at least not domestically. It had expanded so radically, and offered so many products at so many quality and price points that just about anyone in the era of President Johnson's Great Society could gain access to some kind of vehicle. It knew about safety and design problems that led to tens of thousands of deaths. Nader was particularly enraged about the skewed suspension on the Chevrolet Corvair that caused the popular inexpensive sporty vehicle to flip while turning corners.

Today, with the Affordable Care Act ("Obamacare"), Medicare, Medicaid, Veterans Health Care, private insurance, emergency rooms, and nontraditional options, just about every American can find some sort of health care, although the quality varies dramatically. Like the auto industry of half a century ago, medicine also knows that its flaws cause thousands of unnecessary deaths plus untold suffering and loss of function.

But the industries also differ. In Detroit's heyday, the car business was famously concentrated and dominated by the "Big Three"—GM, Ford, and Chrysler. While health care is experiencing mergers and (in some places) local monopolies, it remains a diverse, regional, and highly balkanized business. There is no Detroit of health care.

As Nader found, the leaders of GM cared little about consumers and much less about safety. The near total focus was on profits. However, doctors, nurses, and other providers are more humane. In the main, they care about their patients, want them to do well, and actually do not want them to suffer or die, yet they are killing them daily by the planeload. The motto of the profession, and perhaps the most famous tagline of any trade, is: "First, do no harm." Attributed to Hippocrates, a physician and contemporary of Plato, who worked and trained students on the Greek islands of Cos and Delos four centuries before Christ, we know little about him—or rather them—since the Hippocratic collection of over 60 volumes came out over about two hundred years.

Regardless, the statement which may have meant not to perform wild, unjustified surgeries or drug therapies on patients certainly compares favorably to the most famous phrase of my profession: "The first thing we do, let's kill all the lawyers," which always brings down the house when Dick the Butcher bruits it in Shakespeare's *Henry VI, Part 2*. Still, the Hippocratic Oath is seen by modern doctors and others such as naturopaths as promoting a careful holistic approach to the patient. Recited at medical school graduations, it is displayed prominently on the cover of the IOM report *To Err is Human*.

But the key distinction between the auto industry and health care is in their consumers. Drivers for the most part are relatively healthy, intact, and free to stop or go as they please. Patients make their journeys in weakened, confused, confined, and nearly naked states that make them utterly dependent on and vulnerable to their medical masters, the best of whom increasingly recognize that their positions of power entail heightened vigilance and protection against errors that nullify treatments and ruin lives. This concern is largely a development of the late twentieth century.

Medical errors always have been with us. As Voltaire wrote in *Candide* (1759), "Despite the attention and ministrations of the leading medical doctors in Europe, he survived." But the profession tended to ignore or gloss over its flaws and mishaps. The standard medical histories pay scant heed to errors. Rather, they recount the astonishing triumphs of geniuses and heroes over plague, leprosy, typhus, cholera, malaria, polio, smallpox, heart disease, cancer, AIDS, and other decimating illnesses while spending only a handful of pages on iatrogenic (meaning caused by errors in treatment or examination) disasters such as

Thalidomide, the supposed safe replacement for barbiturates that when taken in pregnancy stunted the development of children's limbs. But common medical errors in the hospital and clinical practice remained very much under the radar until the post-Vietnam, post-Watergate era.

For most of the twentieth century, Americans lived in a Norman Rockwell, Marcus Welby haze about medicine. Doctors were wise and respected. Hospitals were thought to be clean, quiet, safe, and well-equipped, well-intentioned *charitable* organizations. No one expected to be the victim of an error. Emergency rooms all were ready, able, and equal. We picked them by proximity. Every medical school was thought to be excellent.

In *Unsafe at Any Speed*, Nader tried to launch a new idea called "body rights," meaning that people should be secure against callous corporate policies leading to personal mayhem. The term has all but died; however, the concept suddenly seems reborn in certain corners of health care. You have experienced it in a hospital or clinical office setting when doctors and nurses scrub their hands before and after they touch patients. The reason is of course to stop the spread of infection. When you are asked by staff to repeat your name and date of birth, the reason is to prevent them from medicating or operating on the wrong person. When consulting a doctor and afterwards she dictates in front of you, it is so you will correct her if she notes a lesion on your left arm when it is actually on your right, or she says that you take twenty milligrams of a drug when you know it is twenty-five. Hospital visiting hours no longer are limited. A parent, spouse, or sibling of a child or incapacitated person can stay overnight. The core reason is not to make the patient more comfortable, though that is part of it, but rather to have familiar eyes and ears in the room that can insist on aid when doctors or nurses are not comprehending a subtle yet negative change. Patients are given satisfaction surveys to fill out about the quality of their care, including the courteousness of nurses, the cleanliness of rooms, the management of pain, the prevention of bedsores, and even whether they were toileted adequately. Then the results are converted to graphs over time and posted prominently. These are nothing less than the outward manifestations of a revolution that is occurring right now.

What sparked that revolution? The simple answer is cases that shocked the public, expanded the consciousness of the medical professions, and even penetrated the budget-hardened brains of hospital administrators. As in most revolutions or the civil rights movement, some people had to stand up against grievous errors, and other people were damaged or died from them. In varying measures we are reaping the benefits of their sacrifices today. Like art history, medical history is a form of social history. To look into it is to perceive our values as a culture during times of tension and change.

This book can be read straight through to see how the sudden focus on tragedies in the late twentieth century led to the reforms of today, or consumers can pick out areas of particular interest. I recommend anyone about to go into a hospital or long-term care facility read Chapter Ten, "Centuries of Hospital Infections," and Chapter Eleven on bedsores and blood clots, which are serious and sometimes fatal errors. Seniors might benefit from Chapter Twelve on falls and delirium. If you plan on taking prescriptions or over-the-counter remedies, Chapter Eight, "The Needless Prevalence of Medication Errors" is intended to keep you safer. In order to fathom the politics of medical errors and how special interests bend market forces, Chapter Nine, "The Dream and Tragedy of Electronic Medical Records" describes a major domestic scandal of the Obama Administration, and, yes, people may die as a result. To learn how one big state decreased serious medical errors with a comprehensive, cost-effective mistake reporting plan see Chapter Fourteen, "The Health-Care Environment Should be Open and Overseen," which suggests how such a system could be extended nationally plus produce funds for Medicare.

Obviously I am not a doctor or nurse; some medical professionals spoke with me while others declined perhaps because they had a good reason: talk is cheap in health care, but as in law, evidence is real, even compelling. In medicine, data is amassed at great cost, and usually from numerous patients over long periods in formal research that seldom makes news unless it puts a disease on the path to cure or takes a drug off the market. Studies of medical errors—and by now there are thousands—almost never penetrate mass media. Any mistakes that I made in selecting or interpreting research are purely my own.

Due to spatial constraints and my limited knowledge, this book cannot be a comprehensive treatment of its subject. It is simply the attempt of one worried citizen and impatient future patient to shine a light on a horrific social problem that touches everyone.

—James B. Lieber
Pittsburgh, PA.
June 15, 2015

CHAPTER ONE: Mediagenic Cases

In the fourth quarter of the twentieth century, a series of medical errors captured public attention and drove change in unprecedented ways. It was a time—perhaps the last time—of powerful investigative media, especially daily newspapers that combed courthouses for stories of medical malpractice and did not simply report initial filings or final verdicts. Moreover, the victims, their families, and advocates exhibited a newfound tenacity in terms that went beyond their own struggles and spread into a quest for broader deterrence and reform. Inside health care, these epic battles are known as the "mediagenic cases."

Ironically, the cases that changed medicine—and finally riveted the nation's attention on medical error—sometimes involved journalists. The first was Sidney Zion, a swaggering *New York Daily News* columnist and former federal prosecutor known for exposés of the mob, a biography of McCarthy-era lawyer Roy Cohn, and for revealing the identity of Daniel Ellsberg, who covertly released the Pentagon Papers to the *New York Times* and *Washington Post*. On Sunday evening, March 4, 1984, his eighteen-year-old daughter Libby, a Bennington College freshman with a mass of dark curls, taxied to the emergency room at well-regarded New York Hospital on Manhattan's Upper East Side. Her symptoms included a 102-degree fever and mysterious jerking movements. In recent days Libby, who was doing a work-study project in city government, had had a tooth extracted and a cold. She had prescriptions for antibiotics and Percodan for pain. Since January, she had taken Nardil for depression.

The two physicians on duty, Dr. Luise Weinstein (an intern who had graduated from medical school eight months before) and Dr. Gregg Stone (a second-year resident) also covered forty other patients. After consulting with the Zion family physician, Dr. Raymond Sherman, they admitted the young woman for hydration and observation. Libby was not entirely coherent and received a loose provisional diagnosis of "viral syndrome with hysterical symptoms." With Sherman's approval, the trainee doctors ordered an injection of meperidine, an opiate sedative, to try to quell her jerking. Then the intern and resident intermittently spent about two hours with her, until Stone went across the street to the hospital's sleeping quarters to nap. Weinstein concentrated on the other patients. Around three in the morning, a nurse called her to report that Libby was trying to yank her tubes out. Weinstein ordered restraints and a shot of haloperidol, an antipsychotic. Libby slept, but at dawn her fever surged to 107 degrees, she went into cardiac arrest, and died.

Weinstein called the family. She and the hospital took the position that the young woman had a "bad outcome" from a strange and unknown infection. Soon it became known that mixing the dying woman's antidepressant Nardil (phenelzine) with Demerol (meperidine hydrochloride, an anti-spasmodic and painkiller) could trigger a fatal drug interaction.

Sidney Zion's rage was towering, his grief bottomless, and his connections legendary. "Murder" was how he described his daughter's demise: "They gave her a drug that was destined to kill her, then ignored her except to tie her down like a dog." He lacerated the venerable hospital for the hazing of residents that forced them to work for days at a clip and sometimes over a hundred hours per week. "You don't need kindergarten," he inveighed in a *New York Times* op-ed piece, "to know that a resident working a 36-hour shift is in no condition to make any kind of judgment call—forget about life and death."

Zion implored his friend, Manhattan District Attorney Robert M. Morgenthau, to indict the hospital and doctors for homicide. In 1986, Morgenthau convened a grand jury. It failed to indict for homicide, but issued an extraordinary report—truly a seminal document in the fight against medical errors—scoring "the supervision of interns and residents in New York County."

Although it failed to find probable cause for homicide, the grand jury charged a host of errors ranging from callously prescribing interactive drugs to not ordering necessary tests. Under New York's labyrinthine procedure, these allegations shuttled to the State Board for Professional Medical Conduct, which held thirty hearings before passing the ball to the Board of Regents, which censured the family doctor, resident, and intern for gross negligence, but did not lift their licenses to practice. The hospital paid a $13,000 fine for inadequate care.

Profoundly dissatisfied, Zion and his wife Elsa, a former publishing executive and New York City elder care manager, redoubled their drive for justice and reforms. They engaged four lawyers and filed a lawsuit for malpractice and wrongful death against the hospital and its doctors that ran for almost three months in the winter of 1994–1995 and was covered by Court TV. The defense hammered the victim. Dead for a decade, Libby could not rebut claims of cocaine use. The court found Sherman, Stone, and Weinstein liable, cleared the hospital, and returned a modest judgment to the Zions of $375,000 for pain and suffering, $1 for wrongful death, and zero for punitive damages.

For the Zions, it was a bitter disappointment. Once malpractice cases go to trial, only about 2 to 5 percent result in verdicts against physicians, so the Zions had beaten the odds. Clearly the compensation had not worked out. It amounted to a paltry fraction of the worth of the dead woman's normal remaining adult life. The blame-the-victim strategy had succeeded as often occurs in preventing the deceased from being made whole or even from receiving a credible compromise. At the interface of medicine and law, justice often gets lost.

But the Zions pressed on, working for changes in the law and keeping the issues of overworked, undisciplined, and poorly-supervised junior physicians in the spotlight. TV's *60 Minutes* ran a segment on the problem. A fatigued resident, up for days, seemed to have trouble following much less answering Mike Wallace's crisp questioning. An audience of millions probably wondered how such a spent drone possibly could cope with a medical emergency.

Libby Zion's case continued to percolate through the state medical bureaucracy. Instead of ignoring the grand jury report as expected, New York State Health Commissioner David Axelrod appointed a reform panel under Bertram Bell, M.D., a professor at Albert Einstein College of Medicine in the Bronx and a critic of the lack of quality control in hospitals, particularly the grueling hours and lack of supervision of residents.

The Bell Commission report recommended limiting residents' hours to eighty per week. Shifts no longer should exceed twenty-four hours. The report recommended guaranteeing the presence of senior supervising physicians inside the hospital at all times, and the ability of fatigued residents to be relieved of duty upon request without consequences, in effect giving them the same rights a sick or tired airline pilot had not to fly. On July 1, 1989, the Bell Commission provisions were enacted as Section 405 of the New York State Health Code. Better known as the Libby Zion Law, Section 405 was replicated nationally when it was embraced by the Accreditation Counsel for Graduate Medical Education (ACGME)**,** the private body that regulates, sanctions, polices, opens, expands, contracts, and occasionally closes residency programs in American hospitals.

Initially, the Zion law met with resistance. Hidebound elements in the profession believed that sleep deprivation and hospital hazing built hardier doctors. With reduced hours and more supervision, the open secret of underpaid residents as profit centers covering too many patients came under siege, as did the establishment's cherished view that it was somehow critical for a single resident to follow a newly admitted patient through the first thirty-six hours in the hospital. Of course this was mainly nonsense. Residents had been assigned so many patients they regularly were unable to give everyone adequate care. But critics did have a point—with shifts restricted to twenty-four hours there would be more hand-offs among doctors, sometimes with poor communications, and these situations were rife with the potential for error.

For the rest of their lives, Sidney and Elsa Zion continued to strive for better conditions and supervision for hospital staff, especially residents. Despite Section 405 and the ACGME regulations, the system remained imperfect and open to abuse. Like athletes with concussions unwilling to head for the sidelines, fatigued residents feared censure and poor subsequent job recommendations if they left their posts. While a new culture emerged of monitoring resident hours and even sending them home if they exceeded twenty-four hours in a row or eighty in a week, often wrinkles were used to keep them working beyond lawful limits.

For instance, they were subtly encouraged to review patient records and dictate their reports off-site. In 1997, after Section 405 had been in place for more than a decade, Zion penned a column in the *New York Daily News* entitled: "Hospitals Flout My Daughter's Law." Yet, by most accounts there has been a significant structural change. Residents still make errors due to fatigue and lack of oversight. Occasionally, they fall asleep behind the wheel after their shifts. But studies show that their concentration and attention spans are better following the reforms, making errors less likely.

With the Clinton administration's aggressive but ultimately failed effort to universalize health insurance and the industry's managed care revolution, medical coverage in the nation's media expanded. Newspapers, television stations, and networks hired full-time medical reporters, often doctors.

In the 1980s and '90s, Betsy Lehman served as the health columnist at the *Boston Globe*. An energetic, thoughtful, and penetrating reporter, she probably knew as much medicine as any non-physician. She ably covered almost all aspects of health care and health-care finance, although paradoxically, medical error reporting is not among her collected pieces. That is not a knock on her reportage. Hospitals and physicians were the opposite of transparent at the time, errors were shrouded, and little about them emanated from the august institutions in the region.

Often thought to be the nation's best medical market, Boston-Cambridge, dominated by the Harvard health-care systems and its legendary units like Massachusetts General Hospital, already had become a magnet for "medical tourism," drawing over 40,000 annually from around the world for surgeries and treatment.

In 1994, Lehman, the mother of daughters ages seven and three, was diagnosed with possibly fatal metastatic breast cancer. She knew that her only chance for survival rested with an autologous (utilizing her own stem cells) bone marrow transplant coupled with aggressive chemotherapy. Based on her extensive knowledge, she chose the Harvard-related Dana-Farber Cancer Center for the treatment. "The Farber" as Bostonians call it, was one of twenty-six comprehensive cancer centers in the United Sates designated by the National Institutes of Health. *U.S. News & World Report* listed it as number three among the nation's hospitals for oncology (that these rankings are problematic will be the subject of a later discussion).

Lehman's treatment involved harvesting stem cells from her blood and storing them while the highly toxic chemotherapeutic drug cyclophosphamide (better known by its trade name Cytoxan) wiped out all the malignant cells in her body. If all went well, the stem cells would be reintroduced to restore the blood and immune system.

The dosage of Cytoxan is calibrated carefully based upon the surface area of the patient's body. Given Lehman's small stature, the most she should have received was 1,630 milligrams for four days. Instead, a young doctor in a specialized post-residency training program known as a fellowship, prescribed 6,520 milligrams (1,630 × 4) each day. The protocol for the experimental study ambiguously stated: "a cyclophosphamide dose of 4 grams per square meter (of body surface) over 4 days."

Did it mean a gram per meter or 4 grams per meter each day? The doctor-in-training decided on the latter. He guessed wrong. Senior attending physicians, fifteen oncology nurses, and three pharmacists also blessed or missed the mega-error, which amazingly was repeated two days later with a 52-year-old teacher named Louise Bateman.

Betsy Lehman became violently ill, vomiting fragments of gut and lung tissue, but still was slated for discharge on December 3, 1994. Lehman knew she would get sick from the chemo but expected nothing like this, and that day she called home to say something was very wrong. Within an hour, she was dead. Louise Bateman, who was transferred to the full-service ICU at another hospital, suffered extensive heart damage. Ten weeks later, a clerk noticed the gigantic dosages. Disabled, Bateman lived two more years before succumbing to cancer. While at Farber, she not only received an overdose, but her irregular electrocardiogram had gone unheeded.

The impact on Dana-Farber was profound. Unlike the Zion's four-month televised trial fiasco, the Massachusetts hospital simply admitted full responsibility to the Lehman and Bateman families and settled with them. An outside team headed by Vincent DeVita, M.D., a former director of the National Cancer Institute, investigated all practices bearing upon safety and errors. Top management resigned. The doctors, nurses, and pharmacists involved were suspended or removed. Above all, the hospital belatedly spent $2 million on an automated system to dispense drugs safely and halt overdoses and fatal drug interactions, as well as millions more for other safety systems, training, and personnel to guard quality. Other hospitals able to afford the costs followed suit. Unfortunately, after a decade, only about one in ten American hospitals could finance a fully computerized drug-ordering system. At Farber, potentially lethal orders now caused computers to sound alarms and screens to blaze in red: "WARNING HIGH CHEMOTHERAPY DOSE." Plus, pharmacists refused to prescribe outside of standard protocol amounts unless a physician could show new published medical research justifying the dosage.

Lehman was a respected journalist, admired and well-liked by her peers. They jumped on the story involving the famous hospital. As in the Zion case, they asked why an inexperienced junior physician was writing lethal orders, and highlighted the lack of the oversight and quality control that should have caught the error in Lehman's and Bateman's treatments. How could a reputable institution such as Farber lack a computerized ordering system that would have prevented lethal overdoses of a dangerous drug? Was medical arrogance involved? There were no good answers. Incidentally, during a treatment at Farber the previous May, Lehman had written to a fellow reporter that her doctor was "cold and rotten."

It began to dawn on media outlets including local papers in Massachusetts that the error problem was bigger than Betsy Lehman, and in fact pervasive. In conjunction with her story, they covered cases then breaking around the country: a four-year-old who bled out and died following a tonsillectomy, a diabetic in Tampa who had the wrong leg amputated, a 77-year-old who asphyxiated in the same hospital when his respirator mistakenly was disconnected by a technician, a woman in Grand Rapids whose surgeon removed the wrong breast.

Following the Lehman and Bateman debacles, Dana-Farber became one of the safest hospitals in the country. A study from

1997–2003 showed no medication errors that caused death or permanent injury. For over 800,000 doses of chemotherapy, there were twenty-eight mistakes that required monitoring, including a burn that resulted in a skin graft, and an extra dose causing an additional hospitalization.

The wrongly amputated leg in Tampa that received wide coverage during the Lehman tragedy belonged to 51-year-old Willie King, a retired operator of earthmovers at Florida construction sites. A diabetic with circulatory disease, King had his left leg removed below the knee on February 20, 1995 at University Community Hospital. Willie King, however, consented in writing to the amputation of his diseased right leg.

As experienced surgeon Dr. Rolando R. Sanchez sawed through King's left leg, a nurse in the operating room took a final glimpse at the patient's record and started to shake and sob. The surgical suite blackboard listed left leg surgery, as did the operating room schedule, and the hospital computer system. When Sanchez entered the OR, he viewed the anesthetized King with his left leg draped, sterilized, and marked for surgery. Most of the sheets and forms in King's file that the nurse flipped through also indicated the left leg, except two: Willie King's signed and initialed consent form specified his diseased right leg, as did the patient's initial medical history notes.

The surgeon could and should have reviewed King's medical history before cutting. These documents would have shown that all the wrongheaded, repetitive scheduling materials emanated from a clerk's botched keystroke. Despite the nurse's plea, Sanchez had gone too far to stop, and as he tearfully testified later to the Florida Agency for Health Care Administration, "I tried to recover from the sinking feeling I had." At a press conference two months later, Willie King remembered that: "When I came to and discovered I lost my good one, it was a shock, a real shock. I told him, 'Doctor, that's the wrong leg.'"

Shortly after, living alone in a trailer and learning to walk with donated prosthetic limbs, King, with whom the surgeon and hospital had settled quickly, professed to be doing okay: "I've kind of taken it in stride," he said, his crutch on one side and his attorney on the other. The hospital paid King $900,000. The surgeon kicked in $250,000, for a total of $1.15 million.

The medical profession's term for treatment nightmares such as Willie King's wrong-site surgery is "never events," because obviously they never should happen, any more than an airplane should run out of fuel in midair, or a train should race past a stop signal. Other never events include operating on the wrong patient, medication decimal errors, and allowing a sedated patient to fall, among other scenarios whose equals never would be tolerated in most modern industries. The never event suffered by Willie King triggered intensive scrutiny of the institutions involved, only to surface other ridiculous incidents. On February 15, 1995, two weeks before King lost his leg, an orthopedic surgeon performed laparoscopic surgery on the wrong knee of a woman, and then merely moved on to the other knee. Three days after King's wrong leg removal, a respiratory technician mistook 77-year-old retired electrician Leo Alfonso for someone else and pulled the breathing tube out of his tracheotomy hole, thus suffocating him.

Tampa's large and respected University Community Hospital (UCH) now faced a period of de-accreditation by the Joint Commission on Accreditation of Healthcare Organizations (JCAHO), which caused the federal government to stop Medicare and Medicaid payments, a body blow according to the hospital's board chairman Ken Lightfoot. "We do not treat these incidents lightly," Lightfoot added chillingly: "However, by singling out UCH, the industry regulators are refusing to accept the fact that all—repeat, all—hospitals have similar patient care accidents."

When Willie King's surgeon Rolando Sanchez fought to save his license in a hearing, Dr. Joseph Diaco, his expert witness (a surgeon and professor at the University of South Florida) testified that: "It is my opinion that 50—no, probably 90 percent—of the

surgeons in this state would have made the same mistake that
Dr. Sanchez made."

·

Unlike certain other medical errors like bedsores that can be
reduced but probably never completely eradicated, hospital studies show that wrong-site surgeries are entirely preventable with
clear, reviewable communications, meaningful preoperative
briefings involving the patient, agreed-upon incision site mark-
ing by the surgeon, and a "time-out" held after the prepping and
draping. Sometimes called a "Minnesota Time-Out" (because
the Minnesota health department implemented it throughout
the state's hospitals) it includes organized role-playing where all
members of the team identify themselves and state what they will
do during the procedure. Everyone, including nurses, is empowered to stop the surgery the moment he or she detects a problem
rather than tearfully raising it after the sawing starts.

In medicine, power is concentrated, often even monopolized,
at the local and regional level. With little competition or disclosure, hospitals and their staffs often continue to practice according to the values, training, culture, and market forces that reign.
When it comes to surgery, the historical pattern has been top-
down, autocratic, and dangerous. Today, despite well-intended
initiatives in some states, including Minnesota, Pennsylvania,
and South Carolina, and a full-court press by The Joint Commission, called Safe Surgery 2015, disgraceful wrong-site surgeries
still occur about forty times a week in this country.

Probably the most widely published medical error in recent history occurred at the Duke Medical Center in Durham, North Carolina in 2003. Among the nation's elite academic hospital systems,
Duke has performed the highest number of organ transplants in
the United States. Durham welcomed desperately ill patients from
around the world and publicized itself as the "City of Medicine."

Jesica Santillan was a child who lived with her family near Guadalajara, Mexico, where a doctor wrongly diagnosed her with anemia and prescribed pills that failed to relieve her severe headaches, weakness, and vomiting of blood. When she was twelve, the family visited Texas, where a physician accurately diagnosed the child with restrictive cardiomyopathy, a fatal condition in which the heart's left ventricle (lower chamber) fails to fill with sufficient blood to supply the patient with oxygen. After returning to Mexico, the Santillans learned from family in North Carolina that a rare heart-lung transplant could be performed at Duke. For $5,000, they engaged a *coyote* to sneak them all across the border. During the difficult passage, they were robbed in the Sonora Desert and lost all of their remaining cash and possessions, but somehow made it to North Carolina, where Jesica's father started working in construction, and her mother became a housekeeper at a college. The family, which also included Jesica's brother and sister, lived in a trailer; and Jesica got on the transplant list.

There are about 50 heart-lung transplants performed annually in the U.S. and around 200 people waiting for the triple organs called "blocks." Jesica waited three years for the procedure that cost $500,000. Since the Santillans were undocumented immigrants who had entered the country illegally, Jesica could not qualify for Medicaid. A salty, bearded, 55-year-old home-builder from Texas named Mac Mahoney organized a local charity called Jesica's Hope Chest. North Carolinians embraced the cause of the hard-working religious family and their sweet child, whose face seemed to be on every restaurant façade and storefront. Naysayers questioned whether an illegal immigrant should receive a vital organ block that could go to an American citizen.

Transplantation was the medical marvel of the late twentieth century. It required complex surgery on the living and dead from whom the vital organs had to be seized in pristine shape and preserved unharmed until they could be inserted in recipients on the brink of death. The surgery of seating alien organs in

a patient was arduous, exacting, and heroic. Likewise, the medical and drug challenges of keeping the body from rejecting its
new necessities were immense.

In early February 2003, surgeons at Duke began receiving
calls about an available heart-lung block from Carolina Donor
Services, an agency that interfaces between hospitals and the
United Network of Organ Services, a federally regulated system
that finds donors in fatal condition. Two Duke patients actually
were up next on the list for immediate donation called the "match
run." But one person was not the right size to receive the organs
and the other was not ready for the procedure. Dr. James Jaggers,
Duke's Chief of Pediatric Cardiothoracic Surgery, asked if Jesica
Santillan, who was not on the match run, could have the block,
and the body parts broker said yes.

As Duke's procuring surgeon, Dr. Shin Ho flew on a chartered jet to a life-supported donor body in Boston. The Santillan
family rushed Jesica to the Pediatric Intensive Care Unit at Duke.
Since they still spoke only Spanish, Mac Mahoney, the flamboy-
ant fund-raiser and media magnet acted as their voice about the
quest of Jesica, "The World's Sweetheart."

The organ harvest in Boston went well, and Dr. Ho boarded
the jet with the organ block intact. Three times at the UNOS
facility he was told that the donor's blood type—and, hence, the
block—was A. Ho never had been told at Duke that Jesica's blood
type was O positive.

Jesica's surgery went smoothly. The block fit snugly into her
small chest cavity. With a hundred transplants behind him, Dr.
Jaggers appeared to be the right physician for the task. An excellent technical practitioner whose training culminated in a fellowship in congenital heart surgery, he was respected by staff. As a
humanitarian, he regularly provided free pediatric heart surgery
in Nicaragua.

Jesica's transplant functioned for about forty minutes. Then
the antibodies in her O-positive blood began a relentless siege

on her new type A organs. When Duke's immunology lab confirmed "ABO incompatibility," Jaggers wept. He had assumed that the block was compatible. The humanitarian surgeon never had asked, checked, or performed an ABO typing test before swapping out the organs.

He immediately apologized to the family for the likely fatal error. "Duke didn't make the mistake, I did," he stated. As for Duke, it too accepted responsibility but failed to apologize while taking two legally opportunistic positions. It insisted that the hospital and Jaggers were separate since the surgeon technically was an independent contractor rather than an employee. It reportedly insisted on silence from the family and Mahoney while it attempted to procure yet another rare organ block.

As national media descended on the tragic scene, an attempt at cloture left a bad taste. Calling a press conference in a university auditorium, Mahoney alleged a cover-up by Duke that was hindering the search for new organs. Through translators it was revealed that Jesica's parents termed the Duke doctors "piranhas" and "maimers" who should go to jail. The *Washington Post* editorialized that Jaggers had "become a figure both noble and detestable, the captain of a sunk ship, a confirmation that Americans mythologize doctors while deeply suspecting them of the capacity for great arrogance and harm." To Mahoney, "Duke is as arrogant as hell is hot." Somehow, Jesica lingered in a coma-like state for two weeks. It was a new kind of hell at the intersection of medical error and medical ethics.

In the media's glare, medical ethicists became talking heads about the question of whether Jesica should receive new organs should they become available. She already had jumped the line, and had a good chance of dying even with a fresh compatible set. Also, since about thirteen people die every week in America waiting for organs, why should she be able to double dip in the survival allocation lottery?

But when a new compatible block became available on February 20, 2003, it seemed too cruel not to transplant it in Jesica, who already had been a victim of a crushing medical error. Plus, as some ethicists pointed out, she really never had received the first transplant, which should not count since those organs had an incorrect blood type and were therefore unsuitable at the outset.

When it was time for the second transplant, the family asked the deeply chastened James Jaggers to perform the operation. Again, the procedure seemed to go well. But Jesica had had enough. Her brain swelled, her kidneys failed, and she died the following day, February 22, 2003.

Initially, there was even debate about that. When her electroencephalograph (EEG) showed no electrical activity—brain death—Duke wanted to take her off life support. Distrustful, the Santillans wanted an independent second opinion. Duke refused, she was pronounced dead, and unhooked from machinery. After an autopsy, which showed that her struggle resulted in a fatal lack of blood flow to the brain, the Santillan family sought to donate her organs, including her pair of costly blocks, to patients awaiting transplants, but was told that they were too drowned in toxic anti-rejection drugs to be usable.

There were other post-mortems as well: in the media, at Duke, and in the profession. In the week after Jesica died, syndicated columnist Ellen Goodman wrote an article entitled "Doctors Must Battle Banality of Screw-Up." The phrase harks back to author Hannah Arendt's coinage of "the banality of evil" in her famous book, *Eichmann in Jerusalem*, on the trial that condemned the bureaucratic implementer of the Holocaust. But unlike the Holocaust, the destruction of innocents by medical errors almost never involved evil-doers, banal or otherwise. These unwitting killers, torturers, and maimers often were humane, dedicated, empathetic, supremely intelligent specialists like Dr. Jaggers. They were superbly trained and had received by far the most years of education, including medical school, internships, residencies, and fellowships, of anyone in the workforce. Still, somehow they blew it, and when they did the consequences for innocent people at times of great need were appalling and excruciating.

What was the solution? Surprisingly a major part of it was mundane, even easy. As Carolyn Clancy, M.D., the newly appointed director of the federal Agency for Healthcare Research and Quality, a well-intentioned but underfunded unit of the Department of Health and Human Services that tracks medical quality nationally as well as the availability of care by class, race, sex, and region, said: "It occurs to me that there's more double-checking and systematic avoidance of mistakes at Starbucks than at most health-care institutions."

In fact, Clancy was echoing the Institute of Medicine's finding in its 1999 report, *To Err Is Human*. It was ridiculous to rely on the memory of any single person, however decent and brilliant, to do the right thing in a complex rapidly evolving emergency or surgical environment. The responsibility for accuracy belonged to systems and to *all* the people in them. Hence, medicine should look to the quality assurance and error control measures embraced not just by life-and-death industries like nuclear power and air travel, but also day-to-day providers of safe goods, like restaurant franchises, which essentially rely on redundancy, multiple pairs of eyes on a problem, and the mandate that everyone has a responsibility for the final "product." For its part, Duke immediately and at no perceptible cost rolled out a new system in which three members of the team—the procurement surgeon, transplant surgeon, and transplant-coordinator—all were required to confirm and communicate that the blood types of the donor and recipient matched.

The United Network for Organ Sharing (UNOS) confessed to having few ABO blood-typing mistakes in the industry's fifteen years of transplants during which it averaged over 20,000 per year. The agency maintained that only about a dozen, or less than one blood type error per year, had been publicly disclosed or covered in medical literature. But UNOS failed to report mismatches in its own electronic records, and some surgeons believed that there were more. To be sure, legal organ sharing is an opaque, Dickensian, big money system that relies on unmarked private hospitals whose patients—mostly former emergency surgical patients—include only the dead and moribund. Regardless, UNOS also announced a quality reform. Going forward, matched blood types would need to be confirmed by four individuals including two at the organ harvest agency and two at the transplant unit. Participating hospitals had to promise to verify blood type upon arrival of the donated organ and compare it immediately to the patient's blood.

Like the Lehman case, the Santillan tragedy spurred the media to dredge up and dissect other unthinkable tragedies. At the legendary Memorial Sloan Kettering Cancer Center in New York City, the chief of neurosurgery operated on the wrong side of a patient's brain. At Mt. Sinai, where a man received 60 percent of his brother's healthy liver, staffing was inadequate to detect the deterioration of the donor's brother's condition resulting in his death, a state fine, and a suspension of that famed hospital's liver transplant program. Johns Hopkins allowed a woman to inhale a toxic gas, hexamethonium, in an asthma study without clearing it with the Food and Drug Administration (FDA) or thoroughly reviewing it internally, causing the government to close over 2,000 federally financed studies at the premier research hospital. Though no one had died, four years earlier the federal government stopped all of Duke's clinical trials for four days due to safety and ethics breaches, lack of informed consent, and poor recordkeeping.

Another almost unimaginably careless organ transplant blood-typing case soon came to light. It occurred at Children's Medical Center in Dallas, about six months before the Santillan surgery at Duke. A baby named Jeanella Aranda underwent surgery for a benign liver tumor. During the procedure, damage to the blood vessels destroyed the organ, which resulted in an emergency transplant or death scenario within forty-eight hours. Her parents volunteered to provide liver tissue and were screened to see if either matched Jeanella's blood type.

The hospital found a match with the baby's father, who a day later donated part of his organ. Nineteen days later, the baby died and a mismatch was discovered. In fact, the mother was type O like the baby. The father was type A. The error stemmed from the hospital lab which reversed the results, and no one rechecked.

•

In 2003, led by the Bush White House and Senate Majority Leader Bill Frist (R-TN), himself a Tennessee heart-lung transplant surgeon, Congress took up legislation to cap medical malpractice jury verdicts for non-economic damages—generally termed "pain and suffering"—at $250,000. Frist had argued vociferously about "frivolous" suits, and especially a case brought by an elderly woman scalded by a cup of coffee clenched between her legs that she had purchased at a McDonald's drive-through. She won a $2.7 million jury award, which was later cut by the judge to $640,000.

In fact, the McDonald's personal injury was not a medical malpractice case at all, but "we were beaten over the head with it," said Senator Dick Durbin (D-IL). Now, the House Energy and Commerce Committee took testimony on the Santillan and Aranda cases. Lawmakers understood that since those children never worked they could be seen as lacking economic damages, resulting in capping their awards at $250,000 despite the obscenely reckless causes of their deaths. Republicans broke rank. Senator Orrin Hatch of Utah tried to carve out an exception to the cap for "egregious" cases, but who would define—much less decide—that standard? The proposed national cap died, but at least the lawmakers received accurate information and time to consider it before the plug was pulled.

CHAPTER TWO: Hopkins, History, and Medical Errors

In terms of continuing social impact and affecting the medical profession's consciousness, no case has weighed more heavily than the death of the toddler Josie King in early 2001. The precocious one-and-a-half year old was the youngest of four children of a couple in pre-9/11, pre-financial crisis America. Her parents, Tony and Sorrel King, in their late thirties, were an investment banker and a successful clothing designer respectively who had recently moved from Richmond to a Baltimore suburb and renovated a farmhouse into a grand home.

On January 30, 2001, Sorrel's mother was visiting from Virginia. Briefly, the children were upstairs in a family room watching cartoons while the parents and grandmother socialized in the kitchen downstairs. Then there were screams.

Earlier, Josie had been entranced by floating a toy in her grandmother's bubble bath. Trying to duplicate the experience she wandered off from her siblings, turned on a tap, and climbed in the tub. The water was 150 degrees Fahrenheit. She suffered mainly second- and some third-degree burns that covered over 60 percent of her body.

By ambulance, the child went to the burn unit at Johns Hopkins Bayside Hospital, but soon was transferred to the Pediatric Intensive Care Unit at the Hopkins Children's Center where a ventilator breathed for her and a central line was inserted to supply medicine, food, and fluids while she received skin grafts from her own body and from donors.

Third-degree burns are more disfiguring than second degree, but the latter ironically are more painful since third-degree burns destroy nerve roots and the ability to sense pain. Josie's considerable pain was managed with morphine. Her mother stayed with her day and night. At first, Sorrel King was being investigated for child abuse so the hospital staff failed initially to warm to her. Then it became known that the family's new water heater had a faulty bushing. Otherwise, the bath water would have heated more gradually, not exceeding about 120 degrees, and the burns would not have occurred or would have been much less serious. In any event, the investigation was dropped and the parents were cleared. Though Sorrel continued to blame herself, she was welcomed as a valued and avid member of the child's care team at Hopkins, a forward-thinking hospital.

The mother did the right things. She meticulously noted her child's drugs and progress, became medically literate on burn treatments, even borrowed books and articles from the hospital library, and formed relationships with the staff, especially the doctors, so that she could bring matters to light and ask questions. Over the long course of the hospitalization, she brought them muffins and coffee and came to know them personally. Above all, she trusted Hopkins, then as often ranked Number One among American hospitals in the *U.S. News & World Report* Best Hospitals survey. Framed covers of the magazine vaunting the elite designation hung in the halls like icons.

The *U.S. News* survey has been faulted deservedly. For most specialties, non-quality factors drive the scores. The biggest chunk of the rankings (about a third) result from reputation grades given by a small and not statistically significant number of physicians. In a few fields, such as ophthalmology and psychiatry, reputation is the *only* standard. In other specialties, questionable criteria includes the number of patients, which often triggers an expensive advertising campaign that draws funds away from patient care and safety. Another key *U.S. News* criterion, cutting-edge technology, has no measurable bearing on some specialties such as urological and pancreatic surgery. However, the rankings spur the purchase of vastly expensive robots without proven benefits to perform invasive procedures. Patient safety shamefully comprises only 5 percent of the *U.S. News* Best Hospitals rankings.

Moreover, almost all the safety metrics focus on postsurgical complications such as internal bleeding or kidney failure. Unaccountably missing are patient falls and preventable pressure ulcers (bedsores). Worst of all, and completely inexplicable given the reality of modern hospital dangers, the *U.S. News* survey avoids the incidence of hospital-acquired infections (HAIs). These include the notorious flesh-eating germs called Methicillin-resistant *Staphylococcus Aureus* (MRSA) and bacteria from central lines, the catheters that furnish drugs, nutrients, and fluids to extremely ill patients. HAIs, in fact two of them, would contribute to Josie King's demise.

An undeniably august institution, Hopkins is probably the best conceived hospital and medical training complex in American history. Opening in 1893 after almost two decades of planning, its faculty and philosophy merged German scientific rigor and laboratory analysis with French practical training and creativity. Its medical students were the most carefully selected in the nation. Hopkins also was the first institution to require applicants to hold undergraduate college degrees.

No full-scale university ever has been or will be more identified with medicine than Johns Hopkins. Probably this was a result of its early brilliant faculty; regarded as the "Big Four" of American health care, they soon became household names. William Osler, professor of clinical medicine, performed original research on the blood, particularly platelets, spleen, heart infections, and malaria, and excelled at diagnosing and tracking complex patients. Osler's *Principals and Practice of Medicine* became the standard text for medical students in the early twentieth century and appeared in numerous editions. Dean and professor of pathology William Welch identified the bacillus behind gas gangrene, and did groundwork on embolisms (blood clots) and diphtheria. Howard Kelly, chief of obstetrics and gynecology, became known as the "father of gynecology" for his development of a lighted urinary cystoscope, vesicle (small sac) speculum, anesthesia methods, and the use of radioactive treatments for cancer.

Hopkins was especially fabled for children's medicine. As the Big Four passed from the scene in the 1920s, the university hired Helen Taussig, a pioneer in pediatric cardiology, who had been rebuffed by Harvard because of her gender. We have forgotten how many infants and toddlers used to die of natural causes. A walk through a cemetery is a reminder of how common this was before World War II. The author of the landmark book *Congenital Malformations of the Heart* (1947), Taussig worked with Hopkins surgeon Alfred Blalock to make procedures safe and routine, and to radically reduce infant mortality rates.

Hopkins' history gave Sorrel King a sense of confidence. She bonded with her child's doctors, whom she believed to be the best in the world. Staying day and night in the cramped, high-tech, sixteen-bed PICU, only occasionally would she be spelled by her mother or sister. She kept Josie's spirits up when the child had a breathing tube inserted, endured grueling rounds of skin grafts, the removal of dead skin, and the application of sterile gauze dressings. She knew that burn victims were prone to infection, and dutifully donned rubber gloves to smear bacitracin antiseptic on the baby's hands and feet. Like all small victims of extensive burns, Josie was at risk for dehydration and infection. Small children are more susceptible to dehydration through the skin since they have high surface area to body mass ratios. Infections lead to internal leaking from the tissues, which magnifies the problem.

Sorrel King was in awe of Hopkins and thought its physicians, especially prominent pediatric surgeon Dr. Charles Paidas, were gods, though often she dealt with fellows and residents. One of the criticisms of elite teaching hospitals that invariably win all the top spots in the *U.S. News* survey is that famous senior physicians bring in the patients, but junior doctors in training do most of the work, including interfacing with patients. Plus, there can be a slow, cumbersome, and almost militaristic chain of command—from nurse to resident to fellow—that a patient with a problem requiring expertise must withstand before the great specialist or surgeon arrives.

However, while Josie was in the ICU this was not Sorrel's problem. The prominent pediatric surgeon was accessible and provided her with his cell phone number, told her to call anytime, and responded. The fellows were brilliant and accommodating. One young prodigy—pure Hopkins—had graduated from college at fifteen and received her M.D., at nineteen. Sorrel became her confidante about dating and relationship issues.

The hospital's nurses figure less prominently in Sorrel King's 2009 memoir *Josie's Story: A Mother's Inspiring Crusade to Make Medical Care Safe*. In the main, they seemed competent and helpful, but somewhat commoditized and on a low rung in the glittering medical-industrial complex. King offers only their first names, but they played a prominent role in Josie's daily care.

In addition to being placed on a ventilator tube, Josie had an IV inserted into the femoral vein in her groin to deliver fluids. This is the most infection-prone site for a port. Twice a day, to avoid infection, dead skin was removed and a sterile dressing applied. In the early days, Sorrel took naps on the floor beside Josie's bed, using a heavy cable knit sweater as a pillow. Amy, a nurse she had befriended, walked in and snapped, "Are you crazy?" Wearing rubber gloves, the nurse grabbed a garbage bag, told Sorrel to throw the sweater in it, wash her hands, and get the garment dry cleaned. "That floor is filthy," Amy said to Sorrel's surprise, since it smelled and looked clean. "There are germs everywhere, and if they get into a patient, it can be deadly. Not even the most powerful antiseptics can kill them."

On her ninth day, the child was stepped down from the PICU to an intermediate unit. After two weeks, her wounds no longer were being wrapped with gauze, just salved with bacitracin. The IVs were unhooked, and pain was managed with morphine plunged by syringe into her mouth. But it was a delicate process, because the opiates can suppress nerve signals to the heart and lungs, sometimes fatally. Also, the antibiotics that were prescribed to the child, like the morphine, could upset her stomach.

Even so, the Kings were told that Josie could go home in three days. The family rejoiced. Her siblings made cards and banners. But the child had diarrhea and unfocused spells of lethargy. The morphine was stepped down to methadone, a lighter narcotic, and then stopped. Josie brightened and was given Narcan, a fast-acting anti-withdrawal drug. The diarrhea persisted, fluids were cut back, and she was limited to ice chips. She screamed for water and sucked at her washrag. She was weak and painfully thin. Sorrel asked the rounding doctors to come, but was told they were seeing other patients. Finally they arrived, did a cursory examination, and announced no dangers.

Then there were miscommunications with nurses. A temp from an agency first refused to give Sorrel the bacitracin for the baby's foot rubs, and then threw tubes of it on the bed. Another entered with a syringe of methadone. Sorrel insisted the drug had been stopped. The nurse said the order had been changed and administered the narcotic.

Josie's eyes rolled back and she became unresponsive. Sorrel screamed for help, as did the nurse. Josie returned to the PICU, a ventilator, and an IV hose. But it was too late. The child had suffered cardiac arrest. Dr. Charles Paidas, the great pediatric surgeon, now was on the scene, explaining that the cause was sepsis, a systemic blood-borne infection.

"No, you're wrong, Chuck," Sorrel raged. "I was there. I saw it all happening. She was thirsty, and you gave her methadone. She shouldn't have gotten the methadone. It was the drug and dehydration. And you all know it." Sorrel thought: "It was as if she had run a marathon and then a bottle of vodka had been forced down her throat." The next morning, February 22, 2001, a team of neurologists pronounced Josie brain-dead.

An autopsy reported that the child died from "complications" of her burns. As mentioned earlier, whether in a post-mortem or in an obituary, the term "complications" often is code for medical errors. Hopkins, to its credit, performed a searching review. Two infections—one from a central line and one from the effects of antibiotics that had overcome the protective gut flora—had gone untreated, even unnoticed despite the diarrhea and dehydration. Nursing simply had relied on a rather crude but traditional counting of "ins" and "outs," basically balancing between the intake of food and fluids with the weight of the waste in the baby's diaper. But when the child became septic, she experienced additional internal fluid loss from her blood vessels. Communications also broke down. She should have gone back to the PICU far sooner, but a doctor seeking the move was ignored. An independent review reported that the methadone caused the cardiac arrest that killed her. In fact, the drug worked in tandem with the infection, since it reduced her blood pressure and hastened internal fluid loss. Dr. Peter Pronovost, a Hopkins critical care physician and anesthesiologist, concluded that "Josie died of a Third World disease—dehydration—in the best hospital in the world . . . How could that possibly happen? The answer is, we've created a system that's allowed it to happen."

Promptly admitting its errors to the King family, Hopkins offered the maximum settlement allowed in Maryland, a "tort reform state," which was $1.5 million. The Kings declined to respond. "What will we do with Hopkins?" Sorrel wrote in her journal, "How can they get away with this?"

The young couple went through withering grief, anger, and considered divorce, but knit back together and bore up for their children. The September 11 massacre later that year seemed to motivate them to fight against senseless death and human tragedy. They told Hopkins that they would take the settlement, but only if the hospital would partner with them to prevent medical errors. They used the funds to set up the Josie King Foundation, which Sorrel ran out of a room in the house where the child had been burned a year before.

Already studying the epidemic of fatal and crippling medical errors, Dr. Peter Pronovost offered to work alongside her. She was skeptical. The trim, athletic Pronovost looked younger than his thirty-eight years. She did not want to cast her fate again with a medical whiz kid. As for Pronovost, he understood that even very smart doctors were prone to mistakes. He readily admitted to making one: removing a ventilator tube from a patient who was not yet ready to breathe on her own, who then failed to get enough oxygen to her brain, causing an injury that luckily was reversed. One of the commonalities of the doctors who plunge into this field is that they have made and then candidly report a serious error leading to death, near death, or injury.

Sorrel King began to lecture at Hopkins and in other hospitals, sometimes with Pronovost. She stressed the communications failures in her child's case, and how providers in error must observe three maxims: "Apologize. Tell the truth. And take steps to fix the problem (hopefully in real time and as early as possible)." She championed the deployment of rapid response teams. When a hospital patient, nurse, family member, or advocate senses something going wrong with the patient and is unable to get medical attention, he or she can call a special number where a trained operator will assess the situation and if warranted can send a team including physicians to investigate. Such teams were implemented at Hopkins and a host of major hospital systems including UPMC in Pennsylvania.

The Josie King Foundation created a website, josieking .org, with information about her accident, resulting safety measures, databases on medical errors, and ideas on how patients and providers can avoid errors, or survive them. Sorrel King watched Hopkins like a hawk and publicized lapses in safety, such as the 2003 death of five-year-old Brianna Cohen, who had a successful bone marrow transplant at Hopkins Children's Center for brain cancer. Unfortunately, she was sent home with an intravenous bag containing five times the prescribed dose of potassium, which caused cardiac arrest and killed her. Poor communication among the discharge team, visiting nurse, and pharmacy proved lethal.

Hopkins improved, and in fact it became a major center of the anti-medical error revolution. Once famed for its Big Four medical giants, the university now could be seen as having the Big Three physicians in the twenty-first century fight against killing and maiming by health care.

The first of those three physicians, Peter Pronovost, ultimately won Sorrel King's confidence. For one thing, he was of her generation. He had a daughter, Emma, who was Josie King's age and even looked a bit like the child who had died unnecessarily. Pronovost also had had a medical mistake forever scar his family. When he was a first-year medical student at Hopkins, his 50-year-old father, who lived in Connecticut, was suffering from what had been diagnosed as leukemia. Pronovost brought him to Hopkins for a second opinion. The oncologist said that the man had lymphoma rather than leukemia. If he had been diagnosed properly earlier, he could have undergone a bone marrow transplant, but now it was too late. Pronovost's father died weighing 80 pounds and wracked with excruciating pain. In addition to his M.D., and pursuing a critical care residency in anesthesiology, Pronovost received a Ph.D. focusing on hospital safety from the Bloomberg School of Public Health at Hopkins. A common trait among anti-error physicians is a background in public health.

The basic public-health orientation is prevention while medicine tends to react to trauma, illness, or symptoms.

Pronovost's dissertation research assessed survival rates of patients in the ICU who underwent aortic surgery. When they had a critical care intensivist on the team, mortality was reduced by 39 percent and length of stay by 29 percent. Published in the *Journal of the American Medical Association,* the thesis won wide attention. At the time, only about 5 to 10 percent of ICU patients were followed by intensivists. The Leap Frog Group, an association of Fortune 500 companies concerned with health care, picked the idea as one of those that it believed could sharply affect the medical costs and quality of its members' employees, and the use of intensivists in ICU teams in aortic surgery became common.

In the wake of the Josie King tragedy, Hopkins turned Pronovost loose on medical errors and patient safety. Both he and Sorrel King were concerned about preventing "sentinel events," unexpected crises that resulted in death or serious bodily injury. Earlier, the Joint Commission had found that over 70 percent of sentinel events in American hospitals were caused by communications breakdowns.

In his review of Josie King's death, Pronovost learned that a nurse tried to call doctors in to address Josie's profound thirst, but none would come, and the next day the child's heart stopped. He understood that the top-down, elite hospital culture was fatally dysfunctional. "In medicine," Pronovost wrote, "egos kill, and top hospitals like Hopkins certainly have their share of egomaniacs."

With the endorsement of the hospital, Pronovost started the Comprehensive Unit-Based Safety Program (CUSP). The CUSP covering the PICU and floor where the child had been treated and died became known as the Josie King Pediatric Patient Safety Program, and was funded by her family foundation.

CUSP involved six steps, the first being to survey all unit personnel on whether staffing was adequate, management responsible, and teamwork in place. The second educated on why safety was a priority. The third identified local safety threats and asked members to predict "How will the next patient be harmed?" The fourth formed diverse teams of doctors, nurses, pharmacists, managers, and engineers to attack problems. Fifth, the teams got together to share stories of facing and solving problems. Sixth, there was a reassessment of step one.

Different hospital units initially were more receptive than others to CUSP (sometimes only nurses came to early meetings) but eventually all came around. With venerable conservative groups like the hospital's department of medicine, the key seemed to be Pronovost's promise to proceed in a data-driven fashion that would measure the impact of proposed reforms, and discard them if they failed to pan out statistically.

Not surprisingly, nurses answering questionnaires claimed communications as the biggest problem. During storytelling, other deaths and near-deaths surfaced. A nurse in one of the ICUs saw a patient turning septic but could not get the attention of the surgeon, who was operating in another case, and the patient died.

There were reports of narcotics overdoses that occurred when nurses reasonably gave a single extra dose for pain but failed to adjust the patient's pain pump, which continued delivering too much of the drug. Hopkins acquired new pumps with timers that automatically dialed back to the normal dose.

Internal hospital research also showed that patients with breathing tubes had the best defense against infection when beds were inclined by thirty degrees or more, which prevented leakage of mucus into the lungs. Now, simple gauges were put on the sides of beds so nurses could fix the angle.

Nurses complained about "rounds," the historic practice of senior attending physicians and residents going from patient to patient on a floor to set goals and assess progress. Now universal, the rounding process began at Hopkins during the early days when the original hospital building was in fact round. The problem was that the plans were not always accurately or completely communicated to the nurses who had to implement them. Now nurses were included in rounds, as were pharmacists, and communication improved markedly.

Above all, the CUSP teams wrestled with hospital-acquired infections, which have too often cruelly erased the surgical and medical gains of numerous patients like Josie King. In particular, they studied central venous line–associated bloodstream infections known as CLABSI. Central lines are used routinely in ICUs and deliver vital medicines to the sickest patients. For instance, central lines supply epinephrine directly into the hearts of people suffering from cardiac arrest. As in other hospitals, most physicians and nurses at Hopkins simply seemed to accept that a certain proportion of central line patients would be infected with brutal and often deadly bacteria. The national CLABSI rate in ICUs was about 4 percent. Hopkins, as Pronovost found surprisingly, was even dirtier, with an 11 percent error rate. Also, about one in five patients who gets a CLABSI dies. That means that about 30,000 to 60,000 patients in the U.S. succumb per year.

Pronovost set out to prove that CLABSIs were preventable, and that deaths could be virtually eliminated. He knew that there were anti-CLABSI protocols that had been developed by the World Health Organization of the United Nations and by the U.S. Centers for Disease Control and Prevention (CDC). Unfortunately, these standards were dense, unwieldy, and difficult to absorb and recall. The CDC guidelines ran to 120 pages. Doctors simply could not be expected to fumble with them, especially when they had a patient in a dire situation.

Pronovost and his team decided to try to boil the CDC guidelines down to their essence. Ultimately, they arrived at a remarkably clear, simple, and limited five-part checklist for central lines and posted it in all ICUs:

- Wash your hands using soap or alcohol prior to placing the catheter
- Wear sterile gloves, hat, mask, and gown and completely cover the patient with sterile drapes
- Avoid placing the catheter in the groin if possible (these have a higher infection rate)
- Clean the insertion site on the patient's skin with chlorhexidine antiseptic solution
- Remove catheters when they are no longer needed

Even after publishing the list, compliance wasn't great—only about 38 percent of doctors used it fully. But Pronovost kept pressing. He found that one problem was that all of the supplies including the most effective antiseptic, chlorhexidine (which is a non-corrosive component of common mouthwashes), were scattered to various floors and closets. He made sure that all necessary supplies were stocked on carts in the ICUs. Compliance went up to about 70 percent. Then he tasked nurses with monitoring doctors' performance, including giving them authority to stop incomplete, disobedient, and infectious practices. Compliance became virtually universal and the infection rate dropped nearly to zero, with a measurable annual savings of eight lives and $2 million just at Hopkins.

A master medical politician, Pronovost leveraged the astonishing CLABSI success at Hopkins into state, national, and even international programs. A charismatic and passionate but low-key speaker, he saw the good in his audience: doctors and nurses truly wanted to help and not hurt patients; administrators favored safety if they could see a savings. He put provider and administrator groups on the same page with the promise that studies would be evidence-based. He understood that change was difficult, and had to be simplified in order for repeatable behavior patterns to take hold in cramped complex environments like ICUs. He credibly promised that no reforms would be forced on hospitals unless data justified the change.

In 2003, Pronovost and Hopkins spearheaded an effort that included 108 Michigan ICUs, of which 103 reported data over eighteen months. Funded mainly by the federal Agency for Healthcare Research and Quality, the study involved choosing and training a nurse and physician team leader at every site, following a protocol for the daily collection of data, using the five part "central line bundle," including attempting where possible to avoid the standard femoral (groin) insertion point for hoses since it has been shown to lead to infections. The study covered 357,757 "catheter-days." According to the landmark article later published in the *New England Journal of Medicine*, "[t]he median rate of catheter-related bloodstream infection per 1,000 catheter-days decreased from 2.7 infections at baseline to 0 at 3 months after implementation." It was a public-health triumph.

The additional treatment cost of each central line infection is about $45,000. During the eighteen months of the Michigan study, which cost $500,000, the CLABSI checklist saved 1,500 lives and almost $200 million.

With the assistance of Congressman Patrick Kennedy (D-RI), Pronovost was able to set up a similar CLABSI protocol in the ICUs of Rhode Island and duplicate the result, again basically dropping the infection rate to zero. Pilot programs in England and Spain, where Pronovost and his team implemented changes with checklists in ICUs, also erased central line infections.

At Hopkins, Pronovost and his teams distilled what was known about Ventilator-Associated Pneumonia (VAP), a similar and sometimes fatal hospital-acquired infection suffered by very sick patients who require breathing tubes. Additional treatment costs following infection average about $22,000. Again, Pronovost and his team came up with a five-part checklist involving:

- A thirty-degree elevation of the head of the bed, which prevented dripping mucus into the lungs
- Keeping patients awake at least part of the day. Better outcomes were associated with consciousness than with overall sedation in the ICUs, which had been over-used as a management tool
- Daily testing to see if the patient could come off the machine, since every additional day on a ventilator raised the risk of infection by up to 3 percent
- Giving a medication for stomach ulcers preventively, since they seem to follow from ventilator stress
- Using preventative medication against blood clots, since breathing tubes increase that risk

Implementing the VAP five also showed that ventilator infection and complications were largely preventable.

Pronovost's widely-copied and heralded work on these dreaded HAIs proved that they were not a necessary part of the hospital experience. In 2008, he was named one of *Time* magazine's "100 Most Influential People in the World," and also received a MacArthur Foundation Fellowship, sometimes known as a "genius prize." In 2007, Atul Gawande, the surgeon and medical writer for the *New Yorker*, wrote that Pronovost's "work has already saved more lives than that of any laboratory scientist in the past decade."

CHAPTER THREE: Bad Doctors, Newsmakers, and Celebrities

During the late twentieth and early twenty-first centuries, three other types of cases expanded public consciousness of the error epidemic. These were bad doctor, newsmaker, and celebrity cases.

Bad doctors are a minority in the profession, but they cause harm repeatedly. One study showed that 6 percent of doctors caused 58 percent of medical accidents. Moreover, truly horrendous practitioners often have seemed ungovernable. Even if they lose their licenses in one state, they simply move to another and set up shop. Worse, their records have been opaque to unsuspecting patients who trust and hire them to perform dangerous treatments and procedures.

In 1975, a gynecologist named James Burt wrote a book about how surgically altering female genitalia, including partial circumcision, would heighten sexual responsiveness. "Women," he wrote, "are structurally inadequate for intercourse. This is a pathological condition amenable by surgery." In the 1980s about forty of his patients emerged as plaintiffs in lawsuits asserting that Burt had performed the creepy procedure on them without their consent, often during another one of his unusual signature procedures, "pain free childbirth," which meant being knocked out by anesthesia for days. The operation resulted in searing pain, subsequent surgery to rectify the carnage, and psychological injuries.

The widely covered cases in which Burt, who resigned from practice, was termed the "ghastly gyno," yielded $21 million in judgments, which Burt evaded by declaring bankruptcy. However, the case resulted in a heightened awareness of informed consent as an arrow in the patient's litigation quiver alongside the often harder to prove professional negligence/deviation from the standard of care principle necessary to establish medical malpractice.

A decade later, drug abuser Dr. Robert Ricketson, whose license was pulled in Oklahoma and Texas, and had been denied medical privileges in Kansas, moved to Hawaii. Because Ricketson never told Hawaiian authorities of his disciplinary record or addiction, the state gave him a license. During a surgery in 1999 on a 73-year-old patient named Arturo Iturralde, Ricketson found he lacked the titanium rods he needed to put in the patient's spine. Instead of stopping the surgery and waiting for a set to be delivered, Ricketson improvised. After chopping up a stainless steel screwdriver, he inserted a piece of it as a brace in the patient's spine. It broke within days, immediately turning Iturralde into a paraplegic. He died two years later. His family received $5.6 million from a malpractice case, and Ricketson finally was removed from medical practice.

The most striking case of dreadful doctoring in the early twenty-first century involved Michael Skolnik. In 2001, twenty-two-year-old Skolnik was a strapping six-foot-five-inch emergency medical technician training to become a pediatric nurse. While playing with his dog in his Colorado home, Skolnik lost consciousness. When he went to an emergency room, a doctor felt that the seizure had been a side effect of Wellbutrin, an antidepressant that had been prescribed for smoking cessation. As a precaution, Skolnik underwent a computed tomography (CT) scan of the brain. The CT, which images structures at various depths, showed an odd speck on top of the brain. A neurosurgeon said it was a cyst that a simple operation, not even penetrating the brain, would remove. He added that he had performed the procedure successfully numerous times before. The surgery lasted six hours and revealed no cyst.

The operation left Skolnik with extensive frontal-lobe damage, unable to walk, partially blind in both eyes, and severely limited in speech. The young man now had the mental capacity of a third grader, plus severe depression. He retained the use of his right hand, and sometimes used it to feign pointing a gun to his head.

Over the course of thirty-two months during which his parents transformed their home into the equivalent of an ICU, employed flights of nurses, and bore 15 percent of about $5 million in bills, their only child endured blood clots, respiratory arrest, psychosis, incontinence, tubal feeding, and gained 100 pounds due to the damage to his endocrine system. Finally he died on June 4, 2010, after whispering "I love you" to his parents.

They brought and settled a suit for wrongful death and malpractice on his behalf. It was a profound learning experience. It turned out the neurosurgeon had performed only one similar surgery prior to the one on their son. Moreover, Michael's surgery was unnecessary—at most, he should have received a shunt. Perhaps above all, the neurosurgeon had been sued in other states, including Georgia. He would leave Colorado after the Skolnik case and obtain a new license to practice in Nebraska.

In the wake of her son's ordeal and death, his mother Patty Skolnik dwelled on the fact that the neurosurgeon was chosen without adequate information: "If I had known about the doctor's lawsuits, I would have asked him about it. What you're looking for is a pattern."

In 2005, she founded Citizens for Patient Safety with herself as executive director, and soon gathered about 3,000 supporters. Following extensive grassroots organizing and lobbying, the group won passage in 2007 of the Michael Skolnik Medical Transparency Act in Colorado. The "purpose of the act," according to the Colorado General Assembly, "is to provide transparency to the public regarding the competency of [physicians] in this state to assist citizens in making informed health-care decisions."

The Skolnik law made public substantial historical information about doctors such as their board certifications and specialties, health care–related business ownership, any previous disciplinary actions against them, including restrictions on their licenses whether voluntary or involuntary, temporary or permanent. Plus, they had to disclose any U.S. Drug Enforcement Administration limitations on the ability to prescribe controlled substances, all malpractice judgments or settlements, and any refusal by an insurance company to extend coverage to them. The act includes a caveat that shows up in the doctor's record: "Some health-care providers work primarily with high-risk patients. These health-care providers may have malpractice histories that are higher than average because they specialize in cases or patients who are at very high risk for problems."

In 2010, after more efforts by the Citizens for Public Safety, Colorado amended the law to cover a gamut of health-care specialties ranging from acupuncture to psychotherapy and virtually everything in between, including audiology, dentistry, chiropractic, nursing, optometry, social work, and physical therapy. Over twenty other states have adopted similar laws, and they go a long way toward preventing a patient or family from choosing a rogue whose licensing or malpractice problems make him or her a bad risk to provide safe treatment. However, neither the Colorado act nor other states' legislation have made it compulsory for doctors to be truthful with patients about their prior clinical experiences, e.g. how many procedures, whether neurosurgeries or knee replacements, that they have performed. This gap means that the aggrieved patient or his family still must assert their claim in a lawsuit years after the injury in a difficult case claiming a lack of informed consent. This is unfortunate because if the defect in experience could have been detected at the front end—in the office consultation—then the neu-rosurgeon would not have been hired, and the dreadful incapacitat-ing operation would have been prevented.

The second leader of the anti-medical error movement at Hopkins is Dr. Martin Makary, a trim, dark-haired pancreatic surgeon in his forties, who often collaborates with Peter Pronovost. Like Pronovost, Makary has a public-health background in addition to his medical degree. While in medical school he became so disillusioned with the values of the profession that he dropped out to attend public-health graduate school at Harvard. After earning that degree he returned to medical school, graduated and completed a surgical residency at Georgetown before joining the faculty at Hopkins. Makary soon became one of the leading surgical innovators of his generation, including being the first to operate laparoscopically on pancreatic cancer, and the first to transplant pancreatic islet cells with a laparoscope. The youngest faculty member to receive an endowed chair at Hopkins School of Medicine, he also became the director of quality and safety for surgery. Also like Pronovost, he almost hurt a patient. Luckily, when Makary prepared to operate on a wrong site, a nurse spoke up and stopped him.

Much of Makary's research has focused on medical errors and quality. He has participated in important studies that prove that teamwork in the operating room among surgeons, anesthesia personnel, nurses, and technicians correlates with a decrease in post-operative morbidity and mortality. Along with Harvard surgeon Atul Gawande, Makary is a leader in the Safe Surgery Saves Lives project of the World Health Organization. Using standard checklists for procedures in eight countries (Canada, India, Jordan, New Zealand, Philippines, Tanzania, United Kingdom, and the United States) has resulted in a one-third reduction in deaths and complications across these cultures.

Makary and his collaborators have shown that thorough pre-operative briefings greatly reduce wrong-site surgery and surgical site infections. After introductions and saying their names, the operating team (which may not have come together before) establishes that it has the right patient, the correct side and site, the agreed-upon procedures, and critically confirms that the administration of antibiotics occurred in the hour prior to incision in order to block infection. Then, whatever could go wrong is reviewed, and the roles of each participant in a crisis are outlined. Anesthesiology assures the availability of correct blood products and announces any special needs of the patient, such as those that arise with co-morbidities (other active illnesses). Nursing makes sure that all necessary instruments are available and continuously accounted for, and plans transitions and breaks.

Makary has driven the use of Safety Culture Surveys at hospitals to determine if error prevention is valued, and perhaps above all to see if the staff members would have their own procedures done where they work. He is a vocal proponent of publishing survey results and error rates so patients can become prudent medical consumers. He also has identified the types of surgeons whom patients should hire or avoid. Experience equates with safety. In other words, often the surgeon who has done the most procedures is likely to provide the best outcome.

Dr. Atul Gawande, Makary's collaborator in developing the WHO checklists, has been adamant about this point. In a 2013 *New Yorker* article, he described picking a doctor to perform a total knee replacement for his elderly mother, a physician from India. He chose a surgeon who did many such procedures successfully, with a team of well-trained role players who were almost an assembly line, but provided a predictable repeatable experience, and a short hospital stay.

Makary also shows that the surgeon who makes the smallest possible incision often is preferable, as is the one who is uptodate on techniques, including laparoscopic ones. Opportunities for surveillance usually reviewable by videos improve outcomes, as has been proven in key areas such as colonoscopies.

Conversely, surgeons who fail to keep up to date should be avoided. Paradoxically these include famous "chiefs" at teaching hospitals who built their reputations by doing numerous procedures that lay open the patient, and result in long hospital stays, convalescences, and risks of infection, when newer, smaller laparoscopic routes are available.

Makary has warned of "Dr. HODAD," the nickname of a medical menace around Harvard hospitals during his student days. An acronym for "Hands of Death and Destruction," HODADs are eminent but dangerous surgeons with excellent bedside manner who attract legions of patients, including prominent people and celebrities. Nurses, residents, and house staff physicians know about them but are afraid to speak up. HODADs create complications, harm patients, lengthen hospital stays, and produce urgent consultations from their colleagues—all of which ironically have a positive effect on the hospital's revenues.

During the late twentieth and early twenty-first centuries, it also became apparent that newsmakers and celebrities were subject to medical errors. In 1978–1979, perhaps no world leader was in the sights of public media more than the Shah of Iran, Mohammad Reza Pahlavi, and no one's medical treatment would affect history more. In power since the age of twenty-two, when his father abdicated in 1941, the billionaire Shah had been a stalwart Cold War ally, a reliable provider of immense quantities of oil, and an autocratic and repressive modernizer of his country. In 1978, he expelled the conservative cleric Ayatollah Ruhollah Khomeini, resulting in national mass demonstrations that martial law failed to stem. On January 16, 1979, the Shah, at the controls of his own Boeing 707, piloted his family, pets, and entourage out of Tehran. He hoped to find a refuge where he could receive medical care while a popular movement mounted to return him to power.

In 1974, the Shah had been diagnosed with a lymphatic cancer known as Waldenström's macroglobulinemia that largely had been controlled with chlorambucil, a chemotherapeutic drug. His treatment and surgeries were followed day-by-day in the news. The ultimate medical error that killed him was the first to play out in real time on the world stage.

The 707 dropped down in Egypt and then Morocco, where the Shah received state welcomes as well as attention by his French doctors. France, however, denied him refuge as did England, Switzerland, Italy, and Jordan. Paraguay and South Africa offered entrance, but the Shah declined their invitations. On February 14, 1979, a mob breached and trashed the American Embassy in Tehran. Fearing further uprisings, President Jimmy Carter told the Shah that coming to the United States would not be "convenient," but facilitated his landing in the Bahamas and then Mexico. In photographs, the monarch appeared gaunt. He endured swollen lymph glands in his neck, substantial weight loss, chills, rapid enlargement of his spleen, possible malaria, and jaundice that could indicate gallstones or cancer of the pancreas.

The French physicians changed and intensified his chemotherapy. The Shah's friend David Rockefeller brought his own personal surgeon, the noted internist and infectious disease specialist Benjamin Kean, into the case. In late September 1979, Kean visited the Shah in Cuernavaca, Mexico and pronounced the once-dashing leader "a sad, shrunken figure," diagnosed a likely bile duct obstruction (a potentially fatal condition), and recommended immediate surgery at New York Hospital-Cornell Medical Center.

Despite the worsening relations with Tehran, Carter now agreed to admit the Shah for treatment, and he flew from Mexico on October 22, 1979. Fearing terrorism, the government posted 50 FBI agents at the Manhattan hospital, where a CT scan confirmed the need for bile duct surgery to remove gallstones, as well as the necessity to take out the spleen, which by now had grown to many times its normal size. But it seemed too dangerous to do both surgeries at the same time, so the gallstones were attacked first.

The neck tumors proved to be malignant large-cell lymphoma, for which the Shah underwent radiation across the street at the Memorial Sloan Kettering Medical Center. Due to security concerns, he was transported under heavy guard via tunnels between the hospitals. Tests showed that one gallstone had not been cleared from his bile duct, but he was too weak for further surgery, so a specialist in crushing stones through vibrations was brought from British Columbia and successfully accomplished the procedure.

On November 4, 1979, due to the Shah's presence in the United States, a mob once again raided the American Embassy in Tehran, this time taking sixty-six hostages. Fearing for their lives, the Carter administration now became desperate for the Shah to leave despite the fact that his blood counts dropped precipitously, indicating that removal of the spleen (a procedure carrying about a 15 percent risk of death) was a necessity.

The operation could have been performed in Mexico, which had refused to allow his return. "The Shah is not welcome in Mexico," the country cabled. "His presence is becoming a threat to our national interest."

Washington negotiated with Panamanian strongman Omar Torrijos, whose country had suitable hospital facilities. When the Shah refused to have any surgeon from New York Hospital perform the surgery, Dr. Kean induced Dr. Michael DeBakey to take the case. Probably the most famous physician of his time, DeBakey served as the head of surgery at Baylor College of Medicine in Houston. His numerous contributions included refining lung machines and transfusions, performing the first successful carotid endarterectomy (removing the diseased inner coating of the artery), innovating aneurysm surgery, and replacing blood vessels with Dacron tubes (which earned him a Lasker Award in 1963). Probably the most prestigious award in American Medicine, the Lasker sometimes is referred to as the "American Nobel."

Working with engineers at the Rice Institute in Houston, DeBakey developed and successfully implemented a mechanical heart pump known as an auxiliary ventricle (the left ventricle is the heart's main pumping component). In 1966, DeBakey placed the first fully synthetic heart in a patient, but the man succumbed to blood clots.

In operating rooms worldwide, surgeons ask for a "DeBakey," a forceps that its namesake designed. DeBakey's innovations in surgery and in medical tools would earn him many other awards. In 1969, he was given the Presidential Medal of Freedom by Lyndon B. Johnson, and in 1987 Ronald Reagan would award him the Presidential Medal of Science. In April of 2008, just months before his death, he was awarded the Congressional Gold Medal, the legislature's highest civilian honor.

DeBakey, however, was a 66-year-old heart surgeon, not a gut surgeon, though long ago he had graduated from a general surgery residency before specializing in cardiac procedures. Martin Makary, a proponent of specialization and experience as an error shield, subsequently analyzed Debakey's scholarly papers and found that 95 percent focused on heart surgery. Panamanian surgeons familiar with splenectomy did not want DeBakey to operate. When they first arrived at Paitilla Hospital in the Canal Zone, DeBakey and Kean were turned back by armed guards and not allowed to examine the Shah, but eventually they were permitted to see him.

No slouch when it came to security—his hated Savak secret police had dominated, killed, cowed, and bribed Iranians for decades—the Shah felt unsafe in Panama and feared assassination on the operating table. Later, it came out that Torrijos had been negotiating the Shah's extradition to Iran to stand trial.

With his spleen ten times normal size, the Shah fled to Egypt. At the behest of his friend President Anwar Sadat, he entered Maadi Military Hospital outside Cairo, which Kean described as "a hygienic disaster area," but DeBakey remained game. On

March 28, 1980, with the Shah's head pointing toward Mecca, the superstar surgeon performed the procedure in about 80 minutes while the Pahlavi family viewed on closed circuit TV. DeBakey pronounced the surgery a success and predicted the Shah's long-term survival with continued chemotherapy. President Sadat awarded DeBakey the First Order of the Republic. The Shah's treatment and stay in Egypt was an irritant to the Muslim Brotherhood, which fomented riots. Ayatollah Khomeini declaimed against a satanic plot.

For a couple weeks, the Shah's recovery went well, but then he became feverish and started vomiting due to an infected fluid build-up. French and Egyptian doctors now faulted DeBakey for nicking the pancreas during the surgery, and failing to put in a shunt to allow for discharge of pancreatic fluid. DeBakey shot back that he had not cut the pancreas, and that the fluid was related to chemotherapy not infection. About three months after the surgery, a French doctor drained 1.5 liters of pus and infected pancreatic pieces from the Shah, who died three weeks later. Infection was the principle cause. A Muslim Brotherhood member murdered Sadat in October 1981. The care and treatment of the Shah likely was a factor, as it clearly was in the taking of American hostages in Tehran.

DeBakey, whose titanic reputation seemed not to suffer from the botched splenectomy, lived and practiced into great age. At 97, he was discovered to have a serious aortic split and underwent a surgical procedure that he had pioneered long before. It was successful and he survived until two months short of his 100th birthday. In his memory, the Lasker Foundation created the Lasker-DeBakey Clinical Medical Research Award for improvements to the clinical treatment of patients.

Research repeatedly confirmed that specialized surgical experience is the key to good outcomes and certainly trumps using a superstar surgeon from outside the field. In 1995, a New York study revealed four times the mortality rate for patients of inexperienced heart surgeons. A key 2003 University of Michigan study published in the *New England Journal of Medicine* found mortality rates across specialties linked directly to the surgeon's experience. Martin Makary, a pancreatic surgeon, found the results particularly telling in his dangerous field where surgeons who performed less than two surgeries per year had a 14.7 percent death rate; but surgeons who performed two to four surgeries per year had an 8.5 percent death rate, and those who performed more than four had a 4.6 percent death rate.

Many Americans may not have cared for or liked the Shah, but they saw that even the priciest treatment could lead to suffering and death. However, they certainly cared about entertainment celebrities and stars, some of whom were having disastrous outcomes in treatment.

In 1979, Oscar-winning actor and social icon John Wayne died of colon cancer at 72, because his polyps went undetected at Harvard. If his doctor there had found them, according to Makary, "perhaps the John Wayne Cancer Institute might have gone to Harvard rather than UCLA."

In 1981, President Ronald Reagan was shot by John Hinckley, Jr. Surgeons competently addressed the bullet wound and saved Reagan, but they almost killed him again with an improperly placed central line that forced the president to endure an unnecessary open lung surgery, near death, and a longer recovery.

On February 20, 1987, Andy Warhol, 58, was admitted to New York Hospital-Cornell Medical Center for surgery to remove an enlarged gallbladder. The great pop artist, probably the last painter to hold a widespread claim on mass consciousness, was otherwise healthy. Soon after the minor, routine surgery, he seemed to be recovering well: walking the floor, talking on the phone, receiving visitors, and watching TV. Then, according to the hospital, he died in his sleep of a heart attack, which it claimed none of the doctors could have foreseen or prevented. Dr. Elliot M. Gross, the chief medical examiner for New York City, simply reported an unexplained death of a relatively young person in apparently good health. The New York City Department of Health later looked at the treatment and found numerous "deficiencies," including failing to perform tests before surgery and charting errors. Warhol also seemed to have been overloaded with intravenous fluids without measuring his intake against the liquids that he purged. While the cause of death never was established conclusively, the treatment that a superstar artist received in a prestigious institution was far less than ideal, and further frightened average people about what would happen to them when they entered hospitals.

Warhol, who was deathly afraid of hospitals and had often tried alternative treatments to avoid them, died on February 22, 1987. February 22 also is the date that Josie King and Jesica Santillan died, as well as Peter Pronovost's birthday. In the field of medical error prevention, it sometimes is seen as an unofficial memorial day for those who have been killed or harmed.

■

In 1998, Dana Carvey, the *Saturday Night Live* comedian and impersonator of President George H. W. Bush, among others, underwent coronary artery bypass surgery for a blockage that appeared to be hereditary. He was operated on at Marin General Hospital near his home in Northern California and told that the procedure was a success. Two months later, he experienced a recurrence of the burning feeling in his chest that had led him to undergo the open heart procedure. Believing that something had gone wrong with the bypass, he entered Cedars-Sinai Medical Center in Los Angeles near where he was working. In fact nothing had gone wrong, except the wrong artery had been bypassed earlier in Marin, leaving him immediately vulnerable to a heart attack. At Cedars-Sinai, he received an emergency angioplasty, a procedure using a balloon and catheter to clear the artery. It worked, suggesting that even open heart bypass surgery on the correct vessel would have been unnecessary.

Carvey sued Marin surgeon Elias Hanna for $7.5 million to make a point and prevent similar accidents. Hanna was highly respected and extremely experienced, having performed thousands of coronary artery bypasses. He claimed that he missed the diagnosed artery due to an anatomical irregularity that cloaked it in muscle, an honest mistake, and nearly a mortal one. "I didn't want to go to court and I don't seek this kind of publicity," said Carvey. "But I felt this was a matter of right and wrong. There was no letter of apology or explanation, no phone call. I wanted to be certain this surgeon would not be hurting someone else and would be acknowledging his error." Interestingly, in the wake of cases like Carvey's and Josie King's, a movement has arisen among doctors and hospital risk managers to apologize and acknowledge errors as soon as possible, which actually seems to cut down on the number of malpractice suits.

Much as New York Hospital-Cornell Medical Center served the elite in New York City, Cedars-Sinai Medical Senter, which saved Dana Carvey, long has catered to well-to-do patients in Southern California. Like New York Hospital, Cedars-Sinai would commit a significant and widely publicized medical error involving a celebrity.

In 2007, popular film actor Dennis Quaid and his wife Kimberly Buffington finally were able to have children. After Buffington suffered five miscarriages, a female surrogate implanted with Buffington's eggs that had been inseminated with Quaid's sperm carried the couple's twins to term and delivered a boy and girl. After two weeks, the newborns developed staph infections and were admitted to Cedars-Sinai for a course of intravenous antibiotics. They also were supposed to receive a pediatric anti-coagulant called Hep-Lock. Instead, the nurses gave the babies Heparin, the adult-strength agent. Both drugs were manufactured by Baxter Health Care. Both came in vials with similar blue labels. But Heparin was a thousand times more potent than Hep-Lock, and the nurses who were supposed to be checking each other to prevent error administered it twice. Baxter had known about the potential for disasters. Six babies previously had been dosed with Heparin at a hospital in Indianapolis, and three died, but Baxter had resisted recalling the drugs to relabel the vials, and merely had sent out printed cautions to buyers.

Over the course of two days in the Cedars ICU, the twins almost died from the effects of the powerful blood thinner, which turned their blood "to the consistency of water. They basically bled out," according to the actor. But fortunately through transfusions, they stabilized and also cleared the infection.

The Quaids brought suit against the hospital and Baxter for only $50,000, a small amount but large enough to put the matter in court. In fact they were not seeking money but systemic changes. Dennis Quaid maintained that "we didn't want to sue the hospital because we need really good hospitals . . . and as part of the settlement, Cedars spent millions on electronic recordkeeping, bedside bar-coding, [and] computerized physician-ordering systems to improve patient safety. I have to commend them for that."

A hospital spokesperson said that Cedars "began additional focused education on medication safety and have implemented additional procedures and protocols for our pharmacy and nursing staff." The hospital's investigation found that the Heparin and Hep-Lock had not been placed in their specific drawers and that the nurses had failed to check the vials. As for Baxter, after the Quaid twins almost died it finally provided new labels for Heparin and Hep-Lock to make them completely distinguishable.

The case also helped resolve a debate in the medical error community. Some had argued that errors per se were not important; rather, damage to the patient was what counted. In other words: no harm, no foul. The point had a superficial appeal. But the Quaid case, where the twins survived and others like it spoke clearly for the necessity to analyze "near misses" as in aviation and other hazardous industries, to learn from them and even use them as springboards for change. Deaths weren't all that mattered—the idea was to use data from accidents to *prevent* other deaths.

For his part, Dennis Quaid has set up a foundation to fight medical errors. As a patient advocate he has spoken internationally, testified before Congress, and hosted the 2010 Discovery Channel documentary *Chasing Zero: Winning the War on Healthcare Harm*.

CHAPTER FOUR: Our Attitudes Change

For the most of the twentieth century, Americans had high regard for medicine and hospitals. The news was triumphant, even heroic. Diseases and deadly conditions were slain like dragons. These included tuberculosis, polio, many cancers, and even AIDS. Women ceased to die in childbirth. Life lengthened. Wonder drugs: antibiotics, steroids, beta blockers, AIDS cocktails, anxiolytics, and antidepressants made us healthier and happier. In vitro and other fertility methods helped to make more of us. Doctors and hospitals were admired, trusted, held in high repute, and generally thought to be safe. Patients picked hospitals by location and availability of parking, or simply based on where their physicians told them to go. Most Americans felt we had the best health-care system in the world.

This image changed in the late twentieth century and medical errors were a big part of it. Surveys showed patients and providers were growing skeptical and fearful. In a 1997 survey conducted by the National Patient Safety Foundation of the American Medical Association, 42 percent said that they, a friend, or relative had been the victim of a medical error which was defined as a preventable adverse event leading to death or serious bodily injury. A majority of 53 percent felt that state and federal governments were having no impact or a negative effect on patient safety.

In 2002, three-quarters of physicians felt that reducing medical errors should be a "national priority," and 93 percent felt that training was needed to prevent those errors. Strong agreement (60.5 percent) also existed for the proposition that everyone on a care team (doctors, nurses, technicians) had the responsibility to disclose errors. Doctors, however, saw malpractice litigation as impeding the reporting of errors (98.4 percent), and gave limited support to providing public access to medical error data (26.3 percent). Doctors wanted error reporting to be "non-punitive" (92.1 percent).

In 2004–5, a broad study on health-care attitudes encompassing over 2,000 adults was conducted by the Harvard School of Public Health, the Henry J. Kaiser Family Foundation, and the U.S. Agency for Healthcare Research and Quality (AHRQ). More than half reported dissatisfaction with health care in America; over 40 percent felt that it was declining rapidly, and that it had decayed in the past five years. That figure rose to 50 percent among the chronically ill.

Moreover, seven out of ten now maintained that medical errors said "a lot" about a hospital's care quality. Eight out of ten maintained that giving doctors more time with their patients would decrease errors. Two-thirds were eager to know how many times a surgeon had done a specific procedure. Sixty-one percent based most of what they knew about medical errors on media coverage. They expected "preventable medical errors" to occur "very or somewhat often" 36 percent of the time when "people seek help from a health-care professional." Confidence had eroded badly. As the authors stated in the *New England Journal of Medicine,* "people do not seem to feel safer." Donald Berwick of the Institute for Healthcare Improvement faulted the lack of broad safety standards in an article that appeared in the *Washington Post*: "Impressionistically, substantial progress has been made on awareness," but "most hospitals in this country do not have improvement of safety in their strategic agenda."

The landmark study triggered a debate that still rages. The surveyed population clearly wanted wide disclosure of errors, especially so that they could make prudent choices when picking providers and hospitals, or in the wake of a mistake in their own treatment. The American Hospital Association (AHA) and others in the provider community establishment predicted a climate of fear from wide disclosure, and more lawsuits.

"Public reporting is not the answer," according to Don Nielsen, then senior vice president for quality leadership at the AHA. Carolyn Clancy, M.D., then as now Director of AHRQ, the federal sponsor of the study, maintained that, "Telling a patient about a medical error and what will be done in the future to prevent it should be the rule, not the exception."

In 2006, a Harris interactive poll showed that only 13 percent of Americans agreed with the statement that: "On the whole the health-care system works pretty well," versus 29 percent in 1987. In 2006, 37 percent believed our "health-care system has so much wrong with it that we need to completely rebuild it," versus just 19 percent in 1987. In 2006 only 14 percent of Canadian, 13 percent of British, and 13 percent of Spanish citizens felt so negatively about their health systems that they wanted them rebuilt.

Sixty-three percent of Americans polled wanted medical error information disclosed publicly. Fears about the errors involving children bulked particularly large, and about two-thirds of parents in a study published in 2009 reported the need to watch over their children's hospital care in order to prevent accidents. Confidence levels equated with the ability to communicate with physicians and plummeted when English was not the parents' first language.

Most Americans are worried about care-based infections. In 2011, a *Consumer Reports* poll showed that 77 percent have high or moderate concern that "we or someone in our family" will get a hospital-acquired infection. Medication mistakes concerned 71 percent, and surgical errors were feared by 65 percent. Now, "virtually all consumers–96 percent–said that hospitals should be required to report medical errors to state health departments, and 82 percent wanted each hospital's medical error record to be available to the public." On the brink of passage of the Affordable Care Act, far more Americans—probably by a factor of ten—feared being harmed by medical treatment than not being able to pay for it.

The fears impacted patients' moods and behaviors. Over 45 percent in a survey experienced "very" significant distress about the issue of errors, with women and the old worrying at higher rates than men and the young. These fears translated into a third of us writing down instructions from doctors and nurses, and two-thirds doing independent research on their diagnoses. More than half have obtained second opinions regarding treatment or medication.

Plus, we are worried about staff being overworked, distracted, or fatigued. Nineteen percent in a Wolters Kluwer survey of 1,000 medical consumers said that they had delayed a procedure until a date when they thought the physician would be focused or rested. Eighteen percent have told doctors to wash their hands. New mothers in hospitals now add worries about medical errors to their post-partum experience. Forty-three percent report that they are "somewhat concerned" or "very concerned" about medical errors or injuries in the hospital during or following delivery.

CHAPTER FIVE: Sizing the Problem

By the end of the twentieth century, the health-care industry was avid about getting its arms around the problem of error. The news about accidents among the rich and poor, famous and obscure was alarming the public and undermining its confidence in the profession. Malpractice claims were on the rise; so were monetary payouts. Insurers, hospitals, and physicians pushed back with "tort reform" designed to award and divert litigation. Since lawsuits often arose from treatment, "quality of care" initiatives grew as a method of preventing cases. All of these issues focused researchers on two problems. First, how should medical errors be defined? Second, how many of them were there? Clearly, they were killing and maiming people, causing lawsuits, and mounting costs. So size mattered critically.

In 1978, a pathologist and lawyer, Don Harper Mills at the University of Southern California School of Medicine, published an early analysis of the frequency of accidents caused by health-care in the *Western Medical Journal*. These were termed "potentially compensable events" or PCE's (meaning that a jury could award malpractice money damages). Supported by the California Medical Association and the California Hospital Association, Mills and his team analyzed 20,684 patient charts from twenty-three California hospitals involving discharges in 1974. They found that 4.65 percent of the patients experienced PCE's of varying severity.

This was a fairly shocking rate of about one in twenty admissions. Of the PCE's, 80 percent were temporary disabilities (lasting less than thirty days), 3.8 percent were lasting functional disabilities, and 9.7 percent were fatal. The rate of PCE's markedly increased in patients age 65 and older.

In the 1980s, the Harvard Medical Practice Study—formed by representatives from Harvard's Medical School, School of Public Health, Law School, Kennedy School of Government, Department of Biostatistics, and the Brigham and Women's Hospital—assembled to address these problems. One of its leaders was Dr. Lucian Leape, a respected pediatric surgeon and medical educator who had been Martin Makary's public health professor.

Among Leape and Makary's principal interests were deficient and impaired physicians. Leape was famous for speaking at national conferences to hundreds of physicians and asking them to "raise your hand if you know of a physician you work with who should not be practicing because he or she is dangerous?" Every hand had gone up, and still goes up today when Makary asks the same question. However, three decades ago, Leape and the Harvard Practice Study were not looking to cast out incompetent physicians or buttress tort reform. They were simply trying to define and gauge the size of the problem of errors.

The study involved fifty-one non-psychiatric hospitals in New York State. From a total of 2,671,863 patients discharged in 1984, the team randomly picked 30,121 patient charts and analyzed them for "adverse events." Reported in 1991 in the *New England Journal of Medicine*, the study defined an adverse event as "an injury that was caused by medical management [rather than the underlying disease] and that prolonged the hospitalization, produced a disability at the time of discharge, or both."

The vetting of patient records was rigorous, labor-intensive, and occurred in two stages. The first round involved nurses who marked certain records "positive" for adverse events. Each suspect chart was reviewed by a pair of trained doctors, usually internists or surgeons, to assure that the adverse events occurred during or resulted from hospital treatment, and were not caused prior to admission. Plus, the physicians examined the records for negligence. An audit for quality control then was conducted of 1 percent of all charts by professional medical records analysts.

The findings were stark: an estimated 3.7 percent of patients had endured adverse events, and 1 percent experienced negligence from treatment below the standard of care. Most adverse events were the result of negligence. An example would be an unexpected bad reaction to a drug that was improperly prescribed.

In order to reach reasonable conclusions, the study tracked records after discharge. For instance, it was able to find negligence in the case of a man who was admitted with rectal bleeding, received an examination, tested negative, and developed colon cancer twenty-two months later. Patients 65 and older had twice the rates of adverse events and negligence as patients under age 45.

The rate of negligence for adverse events was 28 percent, which varied depending on the location in the hospital. Fourteen percent of adverse events occurred in the operating room, 41 percent in the patient's room, and 70 percent in the emergency room. The most frequent adverse cases in these hospitals were medication reactions (19 percent), followed by wound infections (14 percent), and surgical complications (13 percent).

In many ways, the study was ominous. The 1 percent negligence rate from "sub-standard care" was chilling, but ironically it also was hopeful. Patient management errors accounted for 58 percent of adverse events—half of which were caused by negligence. That meant that reducing and preventing a huge block of harm did not require gains in medical research or knowledge, but merely implementing organizational improvements, resulting from what accident experts including Lucian Leape called "human factors analysis."

Scientifically rigorous and showcased as a two part series in the *New England Journal of Medicine*, the profession's premier journal, and reported by the *New York Times*, the Harvard Practice Study received a brief flurry of attention, according to Leape, and then fell from sight, making a limited impact. Perhaps that was because it lacked statistical extrapolation to estimate the size of the national problem. Polled physicians during the period continued to see errors as not a catastrophic public-health crisis, believing that these mistakes killed less than 5,000 patients per year.

Regional and individual hospital studies persisted that showed the widespread nature of the error problem and also that medicine as an industry was an outlier. One of the last preserves of workplace individualism, it was slow to adopt team approaches, quality assurance, or to prioritize safety.

Although somewhat frustrated by the lack of attention gained by the Harvard study, Leape continued to drive the reform process. In 1997, he testified before the the U.S. House of Representatives Veterans Affairs Committee's Subcommittee on Health: "Why is it," he asked, "that when you enter a hospital your chances of dying from an accident are one in two hundred, but when you climb on an airplane, your chances of dying are one in two million?" Later, Leape organized and participated in a conference with aviation scientists and government officials, including Senator Bill Frist, on "Reducing Medical Error: Can You Be As Safe in a Hospital As You Are in a Jet?" With other medical policy heavyweights, Leape served on the Committee on the Quality of Health Care in America of the Institute of Medicine (IOM), a part of the National Academy of Sciences that was chartered by Congress in 1863 to advise the government on scientific matters. In 1970, it created the IOM, its third institute, following the National Research Council (1916) and the National Academy of Engineering (1964), in order "to secure the services of eminent members of appropriate professions in the examination of policy matters pertaining to the health of the public."

In 1999, the IOM Committee on Quality of Health Care authored *To Err is Human: Building a Safer Health System*, because "errors are responsible for an immense burden of patient injury, suffering, and death." The nearly 300 page report, which synthesized the relevant studies to date, and brought to bear the talents of hundreds of people from medicine, business, and government, is the most important policy document that the field has generated since the Carnegie Foundation in 1910 produced *Medical Education in the United States* under the leadership of Abraham Flexner. The Flexner Report, as it became known, produced much needed reforms and the standardization of medical training, and also resulted in the closure of many sketchy medical schools. *To Err is Human* already has had an equivalent impact, becoming nothing less than the magna carta of the medical errors/patient safety movement.

While now superseded in certain respects, *To Err is Human* credibly sized the problem in a way that took hold with the healthcare policymakers and the public. The IOM extended the data from New York (in the Harvard Medical Practice study) and a study from a recent large-scale analysis of Utah and Colorado to all U.S. hospital admissions in 1992, which totaled 33.6 million patients.

The Utah and Colorado survey produced adverse events in 2.9 percent of hospitalizations of which 6.6 percent were fatal. In New York the figures were 3.7 percent and 13.6 percent respectively. In both studies, medical errors that could have been prevented caused more than half of the deaths. The extrapolation to the wider society indicated that error fatalities ranged from 44,000 (at the Colorado and Utah rate) to 98,000 (at the New York rate). The IOM ranked medical errors as America's eighth leading cause of death ahead of motor vehicle accidents (43,458), breast cancer (42,297), AIDS (16,516), and workplace accidents (about 6,000).

To Err is Human dealt with many other critical topics including why errors occur, reporting systems, establishing standards (best practices), and creating safety regimes. It pointed to successes in other industries, suggested ways to cope with accidents without creating malpractice claims, generally simplified the definition of adverse event (an injury resulting from a medical intervention), and somewhat complicated the definition of error: "failure of a planned action to be completed as intended or use of a wrong plan to achieve an aim." It divided errors into active and latent. An active error "occurs at the level of the front-line operator and whose effects are felt almost immediately." Latent errors exist "in the design, organization, training, or maintenance that lead to operator errors and whose effects typically lie dormant in the system for lengthy periods of time," including such glitches as using similar vials of drugs for adults and children, inadequate numbers of nurses to prevent pressure ulcers, and insufficient or untrained housekeeping staff to keep down infections.

In *To Err is Human*, the Institute of Medicine vigorously maintained that errors should become a great public focus of health care, and that they should be mandatorily reported. The IOM took on specific problems like wrong site surgery and medication errors. It insisted upon a change in the culture of medicine. The era of the autonomous doctor hero had ended. No single human being should be expected to remember and act upon the hundreds if not thousands of pieces of information intrinsic to the history and diseases of the patient, as well as the numerous drug facts and compliance points for procedures necessary to treat an individual. Error was human; it would occur and cause harm with regularity unless the standardization and enforcement of best practices was rehearsed and applied by teams trained to prevent it or spot it early, eradicate it, or blunt it.

But it was those numbers—44,000 to 98,000 preventable medical error deaths per year—that stuck in the public mind. Death consecrates a problem in America and there was a lot of it, even though the figures did not include infections, patients who died from not actually receiving the treatments that had been recommended, and those killed by diagnostic errors.

Predictably there was pushback from the profession. In its "Controversies" section, the *Journal of the American Medical Association* carried criticism from a team at the University of Indiana headed by Clement J. McDonald, M.D., a geriatrician. They believed that the numbers, especially the 98,000 fatalities derived from New York hospitals in the 1980s, were exaggerated and alarmist. They particularly decried that the overall number of alleged hospital deaths more than doubled those from car crashes. Drivers "survive their ride if collisions are avoided," but patients "have high disease burdens and high death risks even before they enter the hospital." Thus, severely ill patients probably would have died soon anyway. The IOM was making unfair "headline claims." Plus, "[t]he message in the IOM report is hot and shrill. It shouts about death and disability in U.S. hospitals: Preventable adverse events are a cause of death."

Lucian Leape vehemently responded in the *JAMA* with an article entitled "Institute of Medicine Medical Error Figures Are Not Exaggerated." The IOM report, he noted, "has galvanized a national movement to inspire patient safety. It's about time." The notion of "excessive mortality" due to the fact that some people maybe died soon anyway struck him, as it would have struck their families, as cold, but also wrong. High-severity patients numbered less than thirty in the study. Leape pointed to "screening criteria" that kept most of those likely to die out of the study, including patients who had do-not-resuscitate directives, were terminally ill, had had acute myocardial infarctions, pneumonia, or had undergone certain types of major surgery. Many ICU patients also did not meet the criteria. After Leape flogged the "excessive mortality" charge as wholly wanting, he argued that the critics missed the main point of the study:

> Knowing that some of the patients "would have died anyway" is important for physicians because it lessens the burden of guilt. Physicians feel responsible for

deaths due to errors, which is appropriate and key to physicians' professionalism. But we also feel shame and guilt, which is inappropriate and misguided, since errors are rarely due to carelessness. Failure to understand this is to miss the main message of the IOM report, which is not the mortality figures, but the admonition encapsulated in its title, *To Err is Human*.

The transforming insight for medicine from human factors research is that errors are rarely due to personal failings, inadequacies, and carelessness. Rather, they result from defects in the design and conditions of medical work that lead careful, competent, caring physicians and nurses to make mistakes that are no different from the simple mistakes people make every day, but which can have devastating consequences for patients. Errors result from faulty systems not from faulty people, so it is the systems that must be fixed. Errors are excusable; ignoring them is not.

Actually, deaths in the study almost certainly were underestimated. The screeners had relied on retrospective chart reviews. But chart quality depends on accuracy and honesty by doctors, an undefined portion of whom do not record their errors, perhaps to avoid peer scrutiny and malpractice claims. Plus these were all patients in hospitals, not individuals subjected to errors in doctors' offices, clinics, or stand-alone surgical centers. So, the person whose melanoma was missed in the office or whose colonoscopy was misinterpreted in the clinic was not included. The IOM had not focused on misdiagnoses in or out of the hospital (where most of them occurred). Leape also raised the profoundly troubling matter that: "some errors are not even known to clinicians caring for the patient. Autopsy studies for example, have found misdiagnoses in 20 percent to 40 percent of cases. On balance, the reliance on information extracted from medical records most likely led to a substantial underestimate of the prevalence of injury."

In 2004, Healthgrades, a for-profit hospital rating agency, published a patient safety study based on computer models that appeared in *JAMA* and applied them to the Medicare data from all 50 states and the District of Columbia, during a three-year record (from 2000–2002). Medicare patients, exclusive of obstetrical cases, made up about 45 percent of admissions. The study showed 195,000 deaths per year from error, or as Healthgrades Vice President Samantha Collier, M.D., put it: "the equivalent of 390 jumbo jets full of people are dying each year due to likely preventable, in hospital medical errors, making this one of the leading killers in the U.S."

During the brief study period, patient safety incidents cost the Medicare system an additional $8.54 billion. Three issues— failure to rescue, decubitus ulcers (pressure ulcers or bedsores), and sepsis following surgery—produced about 60 percent of the errors involving Medicare patients (one of four of whom would die). The 195,000 annual deaths would have placed error sixth on the Centers for Disease Control and Prevention list of killers, ahead of diabetes, pneumonia, Alzheimer's, and renal disease.

If the old were at high risk, so were the young. Like the Quaid twins, they were particularly vulnerable to medication errors. In 2007, a study in the *Journal of Pediatrics* showed that 11 percent of children in hospitals experienced medication errors. Often there is no standard dose for infants and small children. Amounts must be diluted and calibrated by patient size and weight. Especially with newborns whose livers, kidneys, and immune systems still are developing, toxicity is more of a danger than for adults. Plus, children are in far greater danger even when not hospitalized. In 2006, the American Academy of Pediatrics reported that 26 percent of children treated as outpatients experienced medication errors that were potentially harmful.

The surging popularity of electronic medical records in the twenty-first century produced new error detection methods unavailable to the Harvard Practice Study or the IOM when they analyzed New York and Colorado medical records. Mainly these were "trigger" tools. Triggers in charts noted interventions, shifts, or changes in a patient's care signaling a response to a possible error. For example, giving Naloxone (Narcan), an opiate receptor blocker to a patient like Josie King likely revealed an overdose of morphine or methadone.

Most trigger systems such as ones used by the federal Agency for Health Care Quality and some states like Utah and Missouri focused on discharge summaries. A "Global Trigger Tool" was developed by the Institute of Healthcare Improvement in Cambridge, Massachusetts from the work of David Classen, M.D., a professor of medicine at the University of Utah on the staff of LDS Hospital in Salt Lake City. Classen also served on the Patient Safety and Healthcare Information Technology Committee of the IOM.

The tool was global and "longitudinal," in the sense that it drew from all charts and records, included far more triggers, and was followed by physician and nurse auditing as in the IOM studies. Predictably in head to head comparisons with federal and state trigger systems, the global tool proved more "sensitive," meaning that it picked up additional errors and more "specific" in the sense that it caught greater numbers of false positives.

In addition to using Narcan, some of the global triggers included any "code or arrest" (meaning the heart or lungs stopped), a sudden drop in hematocrit (centrifuged red blood cells) of greater than 25 percent (anemia suggesting kidney failure), a fall, a "bounce back" readmission within thirty days, a transfer to a higher level of care, a return to surgery, an intubation following anesthesia care, a new pneumonia, a sudden stop of a medication, the use of Vitamin K, a coagulant following anti-clotting medication, third- and fourth-degree lacerations (severe tearing during childbirth), and a return to the emergency room within forty-eight hours.

The global trigger tool comprised nine general fields to search for adverse events. These included anesthesia, cardiac/ myocardial infarction, device failures, falls, medication, pressure injuries (bedsores), procedures, pulmonary embolism/deep vein thrombosis (clots), and surgery. These basically followed the New York/Colorado frameworks. Again, diagnostic lapses were not included.

By congressional mandate, the Office of Inspector General of the Department of Health and Human Services applied global triggers to a study of hospitalized Medicare patients in 2008. The results were stark. Unexpected adverse events impacted about one in seven patients, and caused 15,000 deaths per month. About 44 percent of the events were likely or clearly preventable. The most common flaws involved medication, patient care (such as giving too much fluid intravenously as with Andy Warhol), and infections.

The additional costs to Medicare from errors amounted to $324 million per month, mostly from lengthened hospital stays. AHRQ Director Carolyn Clancy found that adverse events were occurring at an "alarming rate" and vowed to improve it.

A decade after the IOM report, the medical community was eager to see if the heightened consciousness about patient safety and quality had reduced errors. Two landmark studies suggested tragically that it had not. One, published in the *New England Journal of Medicine* in November 2010, looked at records from 2002–2007 of North Carolina hospitals with a high commitment to error prevention. Applying IHI Global Trigger Tool software, it found no significant reduction, which was sobering, especially because the IOM had called for a 50 percent reduction over five years. The authors led by Christopher Landrigan, M.D., of Brigham and Women's Hospital and Harvard Medical School were frustrated, but still hopeful on a limited basis:

"Although the absence of large-scale improvement is a cause for concern, it is not evidence that current efforts to improve safety are futile. On the contrary, data have shown that focused efforts to reduce discrete harms, such as nosocomial [hospital-based] infections and surgical complications can significantly improve patient safety."

Analyzing over 2,300 admissions, the North Carolina study found that one out of four patients suffered harm. Over 63 percent of the injuries were preventable. The authors used a non-theoretical, practical definition of medical error: harm that was preventable. In almost 2.5 percent of cases—up from 1 percent in the 1999 IOM study—these preventable faults contributed to death. Over 3 percent of patients were permanently damaged, and 8 percent endured a life-threatening injury like hemorrhaging on the operating table. Were there more errors in safety-conscious hospitals since *To Err is Human* in 1999? Probably not, since the fatal numbers in the IOM studies preceded global trigger tools and by almost all accounts now seemed deflated.

The following year, researchers shook the profession with an article in *Health Affairs* entitled "'Global Trigger Tool' Shows that Adverse Events in Hospitals May be Ten Times Greater than Previously Measured." Dr. David Classen, who did the seminal research for global triggers, served as lead author of the study, which looked at three mid-size to large (ranging from 550 to 1,000 beds) teaching hospitals associated with medical schools in the West and Northwest that participated on the condition of anonymity. The study defined harm as "unintended physical injury resulting from or contributed to by medical care that requires additional monitoring, treatment or hospitalization, or that results in death." As radical as it was complex, the definition did not separate out harms based on mistakes or errors. As the Classen team wrote: "Because of prior work with Trigger Tools and the belief that ultimately all adverse events may be preventable, we did not attempt to evaluate the preventability or ameliorability (whether harm could have been reduced) of these adverse events."

Each of these participating anonymous hospitals had a program for patient safety, error detection, and reporting. Each was a "tertiary" care facility, meaning that it received referrals of complicated cases (which in themselves can be more likely to lead to adverse events) from other providers. Harms were broken down into seven types: medication-related, procedure-related (excluding infection), nosocomial (hospital) infection, pulmonary VTE (venous thromboembolism), pressure ulcers, device failure, patient falls, and other. As in most studies, medication errors were most frequent (here, 45.7 percent) and diagnostic errors were not specifically considered. Deaths amounted to 4 percent of adverse events. Harm occurred in 33 percent of cases.

When different detection methods were applied, global triggers found over 90 percent of events, the government's Patient Safety Indicators (based on discharge summaries) found 8.5 percent, and voluntary reporting disclosed only 2 percent (afraid of censure and malpractice, doctors and nurses seldom willingly self-accuse). Classen, et al. warned: "reliance on voluntary reporting and the Patient Safety Indicators could produce misleading conclusions about the current safety of care in the U.S. healthcare system and misdirect efforts to improve patient safety."

CHAPTER SIX: Macro and Micro

Probably the most politically sensitive question about the size of the problem involves diagnostic errors. In 2009, Peter Pronovost and his Hopkins colleague, neurologist David Newman-Toker, spoke for many when they called it "The Next Frontier for Patient Safety" in the *Journal of the American Medical Association*.

In his early forties, Newman-Toker is the third member of the Hopkins triumvirate who seem to be driving the anti-error process. A stocky, balding man with a penetrating gaze and a gentle smile, Newman-Toker held fellowships at Harvard (neuro-ophthalmology) and Hopkins (neuro-otology) before receiving a Ph.D. in Public Health at Hopkins specializing in clinical investigation. He divides his life as a medical scholar into what he calls the "macro" and "micro" problems.

The macro problem involves the difficult task of gauging how much medical error and harm flow from misdiagnosis in America. It is elusive because much of it clearly occurs outside of hospital settings where practice is less regimented, regulated, and peer reviewed. Plus the doctors outside the confines of hospitals constitute the majority of physicians, the medical soldiers in the struggle for the day-to-day health of patients. These doctors rarely answer questions about their methods, much less their errors, and seldom furnish data about such things.

As a neurologist, Newman-Toker is primarily interested in stroke and in preventing physicians (especially those in emergency rooms) from misdiagnosing it—this is the "micro" problem. To that end, he has been among those who have shown that a two-minute bedside rapid-eye movement—or "oculomotor"—exam conducted visually by the doctor is actually more effective than Magnetic Resonance Imaging for detecting stroke in people who present with dizziness.

Unfortunately, it has been extraordinarily difficult to get physicians to accept, much less train, on this oculomotor method, and where it hasn't been adopted, patients sometimes are sent home from the emergency room to suffer serious injury or death. The acceptance of the method has been patchy, with occasional emergency departments using it. Even within the same regional health systems, some hospital ERs use it while others do not. It makes sense for patients experiencing dizziness, and their companions, if possible, to call emergency rooms and ask if the facility performs this oculomotor test before traveling to it. By doing so, a severe, unnecessary, and life-changing—or ending—error could be avoided.

In order to explore the macro problem—the overall size of diagnostic errors—Newman-Toker designed an epic study that appeared in the *British Medical Journal* in 2012. In terms of refocusing the profession's and public's attention, it is probably the most important publication since 1999's *To Err is Human*. What Newman-Toker and his Hopkins colleagues, including Pronovost and Makary, found convincingly confirmed their hypotheses that diagnostic error is the most common type, that it causes the most deaths and serious harms, and that more of it actually occurs in outpatient settings than in hospitals.

Newman-Toker's interest in errors arose from misdiagnoses he saw mangle the lives of patients while he was a neurology resident at Harvard. An eighteen-year-old aspiring Olympic skater fell and presented with a headache, and neurologic symptoms, including distorted vision that resolved. She was told she had had a migraine—it ran in her family—and sent home. A week later she returned with a massive right-hemisphere stroke that left her paralyzed and with a personality change.

A woman in her fifties ended up paraplegic and incontinent from a missed tumor pressing on her spinal cord. A woman in her eighties, otherwise healthy besides some knee arthritis, went blind in both eyes from a treatable illness that was missed on four occasions. The disease was temporal arteritis, an inflammation of the carotid arteries experienced mainly by people over 50 that generally responds well to prednisone, a common steroidal drug. But without it, blindness often results.

The study on diagnostic errors that Newman-Toker conceived contained a trove of information. He and his colleagues, including biostatisticians, tapped into the National Practitioners Data Bank (NPDB) over a twenty-five year span from 1986–2010. Established by the Health Care Quality Improvement Act of 1986 and run by the U.S. Department of Health and Human Services, the NPDB is an electronic file of medical malpractice judgments and settlements. Closed to the public, the NPDB is available to hospitals and state and federal agencies that deal with licensing, peer review, and Medicare and Medicaid fraud. Attorneys in malpractice cases can obtain materials pertaining to a specific physician involved in a claim. Approved researchers like Newman-Toker can search the NPDB's broader statistical data but not read the names of the providers and patients involved in cases.

Newman-Toker's study included 350,706 claims paid by doctors and hospitals to patients and families. It used two key definitions. "Diagnostic error" meant "a diagnosis that is missed, wrong, or delayed as detected by some subsequent definitive test or finding." "Misdiagnosis-related harm" was "preventable harm that results from the delay or failure to treat a condition actually present (when the working diagnosis was wrong or unknown) or from a treatment for a condition that was not actually present."

The malpractice claims base is not necessarily a perfect sample for analyzing or estimating error. For one thing, data from other studies shows that only about 1 to 1.5 percent of medical negligence issues resulting in damages turn into claims. The assumption, probably accurate, is that the small percentage is representative of the overall errors in terms of type and damages. We do not know why so few claims actually enter the legal system—but many clearly are not reported or recognized, and others drop out due to decisions by patients and survivors not to go forward.

Regardless, the fact that so few people harmed by negligence are being compensated is one of the most serious criticisms of a system long under attack for other reasons, both true and false, that collectively produced the tort reform movement (which includes costly and technical barriers to filing lawsuits and caps on claims). It is true that the fear of suits prompts doctors to practice "defensive medicine," meaning that they order too many tests, often unnecessary ones that raise opportunities for more errors. But it is false that the system results in too many frivolous claims leading to irrationally rich judgments. The famous case of the woman who scalded her crotch with coffee in the McDonald's drive-through lane and won a big verdict simply was an irrelevant aberration.

One of the best parts of the besieged malpractice system is that it produces public-health data that enters the National Practitioners Data Bank. Newman-Toker tested two main hypotheses through the NPDB. First, faulty diagnoses would be the largest source of adverse events. Second, the majority of these faults would occur outside of the hospital. Both proved true.

Over the last quarter century, the highest proportion of paid claims was for diagnostic errors (28 percent). These also produced the greatest percentage of total payouts (35.2 percent). The level of harm from this type of error was horrific. Death was the most frequent damage followed by "serious permanent injury." Death in claims relating to diagnostic failure (40.9 percent) occurred more often than in all other malpractice categories combined (23.9 percent).

Even with its limitations, the malpractice data has been found well worth considering. Prior studies have shown that most claims resulting in compensation are not frivolous. The Hopkins NPDB study also proved to be a fair reflector of the types of harmful diagnostic error. Most simply were "missed," meaning that there was a failure to diagnose. These flaws occurred almost three times as often as "delayed" diagnoses, and over five times as often as "wrong diagnoses." Newman-Toker and his colleagues found that outpatient diagnostic claims (68.8 percent) more than doubled the inpatient claims (31.2 percent). The amount paid out for diagnostic injuries over a quarter-century totaled $38.8 billion. Surprisingly, the diagnostic error deaths paid on average $390,186, but serious permanent injuries were more costly. Quadriplegics with brain damage needing life care averaged over $800,000. The *BMJ* study concluded that: "Among malpractice claims, diagnostic errors appear to be the most common, most costly and most dangerous of medical mistakes."

Extrapolating from the malpractice study and autopsy studies, Newman-Toker told me that a minimum of 100,000 and up to 500,000 deaths result from diagnostic errors annually in the United States. We simply cannot know the outer limit because the harm often does not become evident until long after the mistake or even after death. Also, the majority of these errors occur in the offices of physicians whom the patients and their families know and like, which emotionally decreases the number of claims.

As a neurologist, Newman-Toker's area of specialty is cerebrovascular accidents, or strokes. There are about 1.2 million annually in this country with a misdiagnosis rate of 9 percent. To Newman-Toker, dealing with the macro issue of diagnostic error and the micro issue of stroke detection present discrete problems that are less than obvious.

With misdiagnosis, he is quick to blast some misconceptions. One is that errors are inevitable given the daunting fact that there are now over 13,000 diseases in the medical canon, and that they cross borders freely in our mobile global village, so physician error probably is to be expected in diagnosing patients accurately. To Newman-Toker, the huge number of diseases is not a real excuse, because patients mainly are misdiagnosed in typical areas of illness.

He says the three most common, "vascular events, infections, and cancer probably account for nearly half of all the diagnostic-related serious permanent morbidities. And you can look at each one and say okay, we will take chest pain and heart attack, we will take dizziness and stroke, we will take headaches and brain aneurysm, and just go straight on down the line. You can identify symptoms and disease combinations, each of which could be tackled in turn. You can just lay them out strategically in order of priority based on public health impact. Doing this work involves a lot of research with a different focus than the operation of diseases and the effects on organs. Ultimately, it will involve a fair amount of computer support in real time to be less crude about symptoms, and that may bring in data about rare diseases."

For instance, Newman-Toker and Pronovost wrote about a patient presenting with the odd complaint: "I can hear my eyes move," resulting in the clinician assuming mental illness when in fact it could be a rare but reparable inner-ear disorder called superior canal dehiscence.

The actual problem here is priorities. As dangerous and deadly as misdiagnosis is, there is little will to tackle it. It questions the core vetting function of physicians in their offices, and the sacrosanct confidential doctor-patient relationship. It was basically avoided in the landmark report *To Err is Human*, which contained barely a handful of mentions of diagnostic error.

"So the question is," according to Newman-Toker, "why wasn't it a part of the original discussion? I wasn't a part of those discussions. My sense as an external observer was that there was knowledge that diagnostic errors were a problem, but the general perception was that it was probably too much of a third rail in terms of how it would be perceived. I think there was some concern and trepidation about the fact that there were no obvious solutions and that this might be a big problem that potentially undermines the credibility of physicians."

Newman-Toker believes it will take at least five years before we see progress on diagnostic errors. The government's central biomedical research arm, the National Institutes of Health, is organized around organ systems and diseases and typically does not fund such research. He suggests that we may need "a new specific institute which would be best devoted to symptom-wide research" and laments that "the total amount of money that we have spent on diagnostic-related research over the history of modern medicine is probably less than about $10 million and last year we spent $40 million on smallpox research, a disease that was eradicated from the planet thirty years ago."

The crisis of diagnostic errors that kills at least 100,000 people per year in the U.S. and probably over two million globally is dawning on the profession and policy makers. Belatedly, the Institute of Medicine is studying the issue and hopes to issue a report in 2015.

Newman-Toker recognizes that a new consciousness must be built around the problem. "Cultural and behavioral change is hard," he says. "And you know people have talked about Peter Pronovost's checklist as a kind of genius, but it is not the checklist that is genius. The genius is that they got people to use the checklist."

There are about four million visits to U.S. emergency rooms annually by patients who present with dizziness (imbalance and/or nausea) or vertigo (the "spins"). The terms often are interchangeable. About 5 percent of these patients are suffering from stroke. Most of the rest have benign causes relating to the inner ear. Newman-Toker has seen more translational effectiveness with the "micro problem" of his work on dizziness and detection than with his landmark diagnostic study. Using bedside oculomotor tests, some doctors, patients, and hospitals already have benefitted from early stroke detection. But, according to Newman-Toker, widespread systemic adoption of the accurate, low-cost methods again may be five or more years off.

The cost of these emergency room visits is staggering, amounting to about $4 billion. Sometimes the patients are provided with neuroimaging radiation in the form of CT scans ($500 million) and MRIs ($100 million). But most are simply sent home undiagnosed. "It is," insists Newman-Toker, "a public-health burden of major importance that there are between 50,000 to 70,000 missed dizzy strokes a year in the United States, and probably somewhere between 10,000 and 20,000 suffer permanent harm as consequences, either disability, permanent disability, or death from not receiving prompt stroke treatments."

For ten years, Newman-Toker and his team have been trying to get physicians, especially emergency room doctors, to adopt oculomotor methods. Mainly, they have published scholarly articles and produced instructional videos. He says it has been difficult to instill enough confidence in front-line physicians so that they will "rely on their own judgment in real-time clinical practice and make a high-stakes triage decision about whether to send the patient home with no imaging."

In order to boost confidence, Newman-Toker has developed two ideas involving technology that is less expensive and more accurate than CT or MRI. The first is a sort of wearable, portable rapid eye movement recorder. He has developed a prototype and feels it could become commercially available quickly. He assures he has no commercial interest in the project, and also understands that it would require government-backed clinical trials. He already has spent frustrating years writing grant proposals, but has not been able to get such trials funded.

The second idea is telemedical backup. In other words, a remote specialist such as himself could review the emergency department personnel's bedside oculomotor test in real time or slightly later. This too has promise, but the politics and economics remain difficult as a function of health-care finance. A central irony about medical errors is that they often result in increased profits for procedures. To put it plainly, says Newman-Toker, "the bedside oculomotor exam, portable recorder, and telemedical consults presently can't be billed for." There are "zero dollars for performing that test on the patients at bedside, and then the institution loses the profit on an MRI scan, a CT scan, and potentially on a stroke admission," all of which are supported by private insurance and government payment systems like Medicare. So the institution has a financial incentive to discourage that kind of low-tech examination.

In other words, a stroke patient is a very sick individual, and perversely a hospital can siphon thousands of dollars for admitting him or her after a late, faulty, or missed diagnosis. Newman-Toker is quick to point out that hospitals and payment systems are changing and becoming more ethical. He hopes that we are "moving towards a world where presumably someone will get paid to evaluate a dizzy patient rather than paid for what they did to that dizzy patient."

To watch a Newman-Toker video demonstrating bedside oculomotor tests on a model, actually one of his female colleagues, is to sense what is good and bad about American medicine. First, stroke is an extremely well understood disease and public-health problem in the United States. In addition to being the leading cause of disability, and officially the fourth leading cause of death, stroke costs exceed $50 billion annually, basically divided between hospitalization and rehabilitation. The lost productivity and employment expenses simply are incalculable.

In five-minute instructional videos, the Newman-Toker tests basically include directing the model to focus on the movement of his finger from the midline of her vision (his nose) to the periphery and back. Then, he firmly grasps her head in his hands and gently jerks it from side to side while she focuses on a point. There is obviously more to the test than this simple description and the model was not symptomatic, so the viewer does not have to detect rapid or rolling eye movements in the first place. But this method does not seem particularly difficult to train, and probably, like taking blood pressure, performing an electrocardiogram, or CPR (all of which can lead to life or death decisions) a technician could learn it.

The key to reducing stroke damage is early detection and treatment. That an accurate low-tech early detection method, which costs almost nothing and does not expose the brain to radiation, cannot align with medical market forces is revealing and tragic.

CHAPTER SEVEN: The Third Leading Cause of Death

Overall, we do not and probably cannot know with precision the number of medical errors in the United States. Almost twenty-seven states now have reporting laws but there are few consequences for non-compliance, which can run higher than 90 percent. The basic medical text in the field, *Understanding Patient Safety* by Robert M. Wachter, M.D., of the University of California Medical School at San Francisco, states that "from a variety of studies, at least one in ten (perhaps as high as one in three) hospital admissions is marred by an adverse event, and about half of these are preventable."

John T. James, chief toxicologist at NASA, recently published a meta-analysis of preventable medical events, including deaths, in the United States. An intriguing figure, James has a Ph.D. from the University of Maryland Medical School in toxicology and advanced degrees in pathology and analytical chemistry. Before joining NASA in the late 1980s, he worked for the Army on the "toxicology of chemical warfare agents." At NASA's Johnson Space Center in Houston, his duties included "air pollutant exposure to American astronauts and Russian cosmonauts in joint space station and flight settings." One ironic complexity is that Russian exposure limits actually are stricter than our own. Like many scientists, James grew concerned about medical errors through personal tragedy. After his nineteen-year old son died jogging in 2002, Jones investigated and concluded that the young man's cardiologists had been wrong not to bar the exercise and had "engaged in uninformed, careless, and unethical care." His formidable research as well as a proposed Patient Bill of Rights appear in his 2007 memoir of the loss, *A Sea of Broken Hearts: Patient Rights in a Dangerous, Profit-Driven Health Care System*.

James authored "A New Evidence-based Estimate of Patient Harms Associated with Hospital Care" in the September 13, 2013 edition of the *Journal of Patient Safety*. Drawing upon government and private studies utilizing Global Trigger Tools from 2008–2011, and extrapolating them to the 34,400,000 hospital admissions in 2007, James came up with a new annual range of error deaths: 210,000 to 440,000.

Four hundred thousand amounts to roughly one out of six of the 2.5 million annual American deaths. Even at the low end of the range, this count would place medical error mortality third, behind "diseases of heart" (596,399) and "malignant neoplasms" e.g. cancer (575,313), and ahead of "chronic lower respiratory disease" (143,382) in the National Vital Statistics Reports for the Centers for Disease Control and Prevention.

According to James, now is the time to let go of the figure of 98,000 arrived at by the IOM in *To Err is Human*. Lucian Leape, David Classen, and Martin Makary concurred due to the increased accuracy of trigger tools. The American Hospital Association reacted and urged staying with the 1999 number because it used a larger sample of patient charts. But this was clearly a wrong conclusion. In fact, as James points out, his range may be low. It fails to address outpatient deaths, and the quality of medical records including the electronic ones is far from perfect. According to James, records rarely capture errors of omission unless they become fairly obvious, such as a cardiac patient discharged without a prescription for a beta blocker who then suffers a fatal heart attack. Errors of commission, however, can be picked up rather well. James cited the example of the late Congressman John Murtha, who died following gallbladder surgery when his intestine was "nicked," spewed waste, and caused him to develop a fatal infection.

The electronic charts and trigger tools clearly caught more flaws than the IOM had found a decade earlier. Questions now arise about whether the number of medical errors is rising, falling, or staying put. David Newman-Toker finds it hard to answer but feels that the numerical rise since *To Err is Human* results from improved "ascertainment" through triggers. But John James is concerned that "increased production demands in cost-driven institutions may increase the risk of potential adverse events." He rued the high rates of "fatigue and burnout" among physicians and staff, and that patients must "bounce around in a complex maze of providers . . . in this rapidly changing, and poorly integrated industry."

Perhaps the harshest critic of the error environment, William Charney, M.D., is the former safety officer at the Jewish General Hospital in Montreal, director of environmental health at the Department of Health in San Francisco, and was a safety coordinator for the State of Washington Hospital Association. "Medical errors," Charney claimed, "have become the leading cause of death to Americans, exceeding heart disease and cancer with over 800,000 deaths attributed to error."

Charney counts patient deaths from errors of omission and commission but also rolls public-health metrics into his equation. For instance, he cites hospital research that every patient above a one-to-four nurse–patient ratio raises mortality by 7 percent. Staffing levels of housekeepers also affects death from hospital-acquired infections. He believes that things are even getting worse, including from the trend toward for-profit hospitals that some studies have shown have less staffing, shorter patient stay lengths, an overall 6 percent higher rate of mortality, and a 9 percent higher death rate in perinatal departments.

Charney faults systemic issues: staff fatigue, injury, and turnover are common. One in ten health-care employees applies for worker's compensation. "And," he says, "when you injure a health-care worker you have a downstream negative effect." Bullying is rampant in the rigidly ranked provider subculture. "It lowers cognitive capacity . . . each time a health care worker gets bullied they lose their ability to do the job."

Cleaning time in rooms is going down with predictable increases in infections. Prior to 1970, Charney maintains that hospitals did not merely clean but tested surfaces for infectious material. Then "the CDC and American Hospital Association advised them to stop." MRSA infections since have increased thirty-two-fold. Charney also chastises hospitals for having MRSA contamination in supply cabinets and for using EKG wires and blood pressure cuffs that have not been cleaned. A recent British report showed that one third of pressure cuffs contained the bacteria *Clostridium difficile* (or *C. diff.*) that can cause a raging gut infection if it gets into the patient's mouth.

A twenty-hospital study of patient rooms in Connecticut, Massachusetts, and Washington found that over half of the surfaces that should have been sanitized were not. In a 2012 article, Charney blamed the error epidemic on financial motives and "administrative evil." Hospitals, he offered in a recent interview, "are literally getting away with murder."

Summing studies, Peter Pronovost, the successor to Lucian Leape as the national leader in the anti-error field, told me that there are over a half-million deaths from medical errors, including 100,000 hospital-acquired infections, 100,000 blood clots, 120,000 teamwork failures, 150,000 cases of sepsis, 100,000 diagnostic errors, and 70,000 decubitus (pressure) ulcers.

"It's easily the third-leading cause of death," Pronovost said. If he had placed diagnostic errors at the outer range of Newman-Toker's estimate, then his overall estimate of error deaths would have equaled Charney's.

Naturally, there is plenty of discouragement about the size of the problem. This is especially true about Christopher Landrigan's longitudinal five-year study of the North Carolina hospitals, where a premium had been placed on safety but error rates did not shrink. David Chassin, the global trigger pioneer, who enabled a more accurate perception of the problem to take hold, actually is not discouraged.

"Right now," he says, "we're involved in studies of this with EMRs [electronic medical records] where we're not only working at preventability but mitigability and ameliorability. As we move into the electronic era, we should expand the discussion from its sole focus on preventability to include mitigation and amelioration." He cites an experiment at LDS hospital where 70 percent of adverse drug events were prevented in real time review." So, there is great hope around the idea of instantaneous electronic and/or human review of decisions principally in regard to medications and diagnosis.

Central-line infection controls by Pronovost have been put in place in a partnership involving the American Hospital Association, and state hospital associations. "These infections are down by over 40 percent," Pronovost reported to a conference at Hopkins in 2013 mainly involving nurses. "It's a remarkable performance. And now over 1,200 hospitals have a rate of infection that just five years ago was deemed unattainable." Great leaps forward (as will be shown in later chapters) also have occurred resulting from disclosure and teamwork.

The amount of misery and carnage resulting from medical errors, which Pronovost calls "the invisible cause of death," is staggering. But the leading causes of mortality—heart disease and cancer—combined for 47 percent of the deaths in the United States in 2011. Yet, lay people now know a great deal about them. These diseases have been the foci of intense research, education, and prevention. Think smoking, diet, and exercise. As a result, heart disease mortality actually has shown "a steady decline," according to the Centers for Disease Control and Prevention National Vital Statistics Reports since 1989, and "cancer mortality began to decline in the early 1990s." Other major killers, including stroke and Alzheimer's disease also have decreased. Clearly the time has come to expose the mortal menace of medical errors, raise its profile, and step up the concerted attack on it. Perhaps above all, that includes broadening the use of what has been shown to work to prevent this damage in various heath care settings, and that forms the next part of this book.

CHAPTER EIGHT: The Needless Prevalence of Medication Errors

While wrong-site and wrong-patient surgeries and infections garner the most patient fear, medication errors are far and away the most common—and preventable—flaws in the health-care system.

That medication errors predominate is not surprising. The U.S. is awash in prescription drugs and biologicals—currently we have over 10,000 of those. Plus there are more than 300,000 over-the-counter pills, serums, herbs, supplements, stimulants, nutraceuticals, and other nostrums available, all of which can be misused, mismatched, ignored, or confused.

Unlike at pharmacies, supermarkets, health-food stores, hotel gift shops, gas stations, newsstands, and vending machines where people can buy as many and as much of these remedies as they like, patients in hospitals consume medicines under monitored conditions. Yet hospitals are rife with medication errors. Studies show that about 5 to 10 percent of hospital patients experience an adverse drug event (ADE), which means harm due to an error or side effect. Another 5 to 10 percent have a potential ADE, which indicates that they were prescribed the wrong medication or dose, but someone noticed in time to prevent ingestion.

While the received knowledge in health care is that one out of every twenty hospital patients experiences an ADE, less is known about medication errors among outpatients under a doctor's care, but it appears that their safety may be at greater risk. A 2003 study in the *New England Journal of Medicine* followed a large group of outpatients taking a wide variety of medications. During a period of only three months, fully one in four patients experienced an ADE, some of which were quite serious.

Generally, the sickest, or at least the most acutely ill, patients are in hospitals. They become especially vulnerable to interactive or dosage errors when taking high-risk medications like the blood thinners Coumadin and Heparin, or insulin. In a Medicare study, one of seven hospitalized patients taking Coumadin endured an ADE.

One of the most frightening studies of ADEs was led by David Classen at LDS Hospital in Salt Lake City that appeared in the *Journal of the American Medical Association* in 1997. The survey used trigger tools and employed the World Health Organization rubric that an ADE is "noxious and unintended, and occurs at doses used in human prophylaxis, diagnosis, therapy, or modification of psychological functions." It excluded failure of treatment, poisonings, and intentional overdoses. Extrapolating to the national hospitalized population, the Classen group found that lethal ADEs were involved in about one out of 300 hospitalizations.

While there is no similar study of ADE death among outpatients, it may be that the figure could be even higher since prescribing in doctor's offices and clinics leads to patients using pills and serums with whatever else is in their medicine chests. Homes are looser and less scrutinized settings than hospitals.

However, that may not be an accurate assumption, because if people are ambulatory and not terribly ill, they simply may excrete the toxins and go on with their lives. Plus, when there are complications, healthier people are less likely to die. But to some extent the premise that outpatients are safer or at least less likely to be harmed or killed by medication errors may be shifting in the Affordable Care Act era.

This is because forcing insurance companies—who long have been players in care decisions—to cover everyone, including those with illnesses and preexisting conditions, has stepped up a practice called "steering." The payment policies of carriers steer sicker and sicker patients away from care in hospitals and emergency rooms and toward less costly outpatient alternatives like free-standing urgent care and one-day surgical settings where errors are more likely than in hospitals.

Regardless, there have been and will be a ton of medication errors. In all, reportedly a million medication errors occur annually in the United States that cost over $21 billion in terms of additional treatment and lost productivity.

When and how do medication errors happen? Researchers have broken the process down into four key stages: ordering, transcribing, dispensing, and administration.

Ordering, the initial step, occurs when a doctor chooses a pill, drip, device, or treatment such as radiation and sets the correct dosage. This is far and away the most dangerous phase in the medication process; it accounts for 56 percent of errors. The second step, transcribing, involves the doctor reducing his order to writing by hand, dictation, or computer. It accounts for about 6 percent of errors. The third step, dispensing, means that a pharmacist reads the order or prescription and fills it. Administration, the final step and the one we all experience, occurs when a patient takes pills or receives medication through a syringe, intravenous line, or catheter. Outpatients mainly administer their own medications. In hospitals, nurses oversee this function, and depending on the condition of the person in bed, sometimes perform it.

Why is ordering so hazardous? One reason is that a physician is not a universal genius who knows every drug, side effect, and dangerous interaction. Another is that he or she lacks total understanding of a patient's conditions, diseases, habits, diet, allergies, plus all of the medications—both prescribed and over-the-counter—herbs, supplements, and even other people's pills that they might take.

Today, most hospital orders have been reduced to electronic form. Doctors in private practice can receive substantial subsidies from the U.S. Department of Health and Human Services to convert paper processes to electronic medical records. But a recent study of doctors in ambulatory care centers showed that less than a third had fully made the switch to paperless prescribing.

Unclear written prescriptions are a notorious cause of errors, and fortunately their time is passing, albeit slowly. It will be many years until they are extinct, so their flaws should be addressed. A notoriously bad "script" taught to health-care professionals is presented below:

MEDICAL CENTER HOSPITAL

500 - 600 W 4TH STREET   ODESSA, TEXAS   Ph 333 7111

FOR ___Vazquez Ramon___   AGE ___

ADDRESS _____   DATE 6/23/95

Elavil 20 mg   # 120 -
20 mg P.O. Q6h×m

NO REFILLS ☐

Ferrous Sulfate 300mg   # 100
REFILLS   300mg P.O. TID c meals

LABEL ☐   Humulin N
30 units SQ Q___.
Ram/Galb

PRODUCT SELECTION PERMITTED   DISPENSE AS WRITTEN

D.E.A. #

Ramon Vasquez, a middle-aged man suffering chest pain, received it from his physician in Odessa, Texas in 1995. When a large class of hospitalists (doctors who treat only in-patients) was asked what was the first medication listed, half thought it was Plendil, a calcium channel blocker that relaxes vessels in the heart, so blood can flow more easily, which reduces episodes of angina (chest pain). About a third picked Isordil, a nitrate (salt of nitric acid) used to treat angina and high blood pressure. The rest guessed Zestril, an enzyme inhibitor that treats heart failure and high blood pressure.

Ramon Vasquez's physician wanted him to receive Isordil pills in a normal dosage of 20 milligrams (mg) by mouth (PO) six times per day (Q). Like half the hospitalists, his pharmacist picked 20 milligrams of oral Plendil six times per day. However, the usual Plendil dose is 10 milligrams daily. The twelve-fold overdose resulted in heart failure, extreme low blood pressure, and Vasquez's death within a week.

The Vasquez case and thousands of others like it point to proven ways to avoid ordering and prescription errors in or out of the hospital. Obviously, no patient should be prescribed a lethal overdose of a drug. Every patient or his representative must understand the correct dosage and method of taking it. Every patient should have all of his allergies, illnesses, and existing medications considered for dangerous interactions with whatever substance the physician intends to prescribe. Naturally, this is easier said than done. Of course, it requires money and a learning curve, especially when electronic reforms are adopted.

Handwritten prescriptions—those dread, opaque medical antiques—to some extent may be getting better, or at least not currently causing a huge number of errors. One reason is laws or regulations in many states that require records, including orders, to be written legibly and to completely reflect treatment.

These laws lack teeth in the form of penalties or payments to patients. But providers know about them and fear them, because the violation of such a measure can lead to a judgment for the plaintiff in a malpractice case.

Nevertheless, prescriptions can be made clearer and safer, which is the focus of a movement within the medical profession. Most prescription forms lack the double-checking and redundancies that deter errors in other areas of medicine, such as repeatedly asking the surgical patient his name and date of birth to ensure that he is the right patient. If Ramon Vasquez's physician had been compelled to write out and then print again the medication and dosage on the prescription form, in the same way that the dollars and cents amount appears twice on a bank check, the pharmacist might not have made a fatal guess.

Handwritten bank checks also are yielding gradually to electronic applications, but not because of errors. Some banks go years without passing out too much or too little money because of the redundancy embedded in checks. It seems ridiculous that the same sort of mundane protection is not used to prevent pharmacies from dispensing wrong drugs and dosages.

Another archaic and easily corrected flaw in orders is abbreviations from Latin, Greek, and occasionally French that are inscrutable to the average layperson. This is important because patients come home from the physician's office, hospital, or pharmacy unclear about dosages and take incorrect numbers of pills at the wrong times, which reduces the efficacy of the medicine and makes consumers sicker.

There are hundreds of medical abbreviations; a sample that routinely show up in orders and prescriptions appears on the following page:

Abbreviation	Meaning	Abbreviation	Meaning
a.c.	before meals	*p.r.n.*	as needed
a.m.	morning	*p.r.*	by rectum
b.i.d.	twice a day	*q.d.*	every day
b.i.w.	twice a week	*q.i.d.*	four times a day
c.	with	*q.o.d.*	every other day
i.m.	intramuscular	*s.*	without
i.v.	intravenous	*sl*	sublingual
n.p.o.	nothing by mouth	*t.i.d.*	three times a day
o.d.	every day	*top*	topically
o.m.	every morning	*w/*	with
o.n.	every night	*w/o*	without
p.c.	after meals	*hs*	at bedtime
p.o.	by mouth		

Some of these are readily and dangerously confused, such as q.i.d., *quater in die*, meaning four times a day and q.d., *quotidie*, signifying every day. A few, now rarely used, like "no." (the short form of *numero*, meaning number), "LD" (lethal dose), and "liq" (*liquor*) meaning fluid, are notorious troublemakers. Due to the modern movement away from abbreviations, patients increasingly receive prescriptions and pill bottle labels in plain language that direct them to take the medicine *twice a day* rather than "b.i.d." (*bis in die*) and *before meals* instead of "a.c." (*ante cibum*).

In 2004, the Joint Commission published a "Do Not Use List" of high-risk abbreviations that should be banned:

Official "Do Not Use" List[1]

Do not use: U (unit)
Potential problem: Mistaken for "O" (zero), the number "4" (four) or "cc"
Use Instead: Write "unit"

Do not use: IU (International Unit)
Potential problem: Mistaken for IV (intravenous) or the number 10 (ten)
Use Instead: Write "International Unit"

Do not use: Q.D., QD, q.d., qd (daily)
Potential problem: Mistaken for each other
Use Instead: Write "daily"

Do not use: Q.O.D., QOD, q.o.d., qod (every other day)
Potential problem: Period after the "Q" mistaken for "I"
Use Instead: Write "every other day"

Do not use: Trailing zero (X.0 mg)*
Potential problem: Decimal point is missed.
Use Instead: Write "X mg"

Do not use: Lack of leading zero (.X mg)
Potential problem: Decimal point is missed.
Use Instead: Write "0.X mg"

Do not use: MS
Potential problem: Can mean morphine sulfate or magnesium sulfate
Use Instead: Write "morphine sulfate" or "magnesium sulfate"

Do not use: MSO_4 and $MgSO_4$
Potential problem: Confused for one another
Use Instead: Write "morphine sulfate" or "magnesium sulfate"

---

[1]Applies to all orders and all medication-related documentation that is handwritten (including free-text computer entry) or on pre-printed forms.

*Exception: A "trailing zero" may be used only where required to demonstrate the level of precision of the value being reported, such as for laboratory results, imaging studies that report size of lesions, or catheter/tube sizes. It may not be used in medication orders or other medication-related documentation.

Source: http://www.jointcommission.org/assets/1/18/dnu_list.pdf

Equally interesting are the quantitative reforms of adding a "leading zero" as in "0.5 mg" instead of ".5 mg" or removing the "trailing zero" as in "5 mg" instead of "5.0 mg," which deter decimal errors.

Another chronic source of mistakes are Look-Alike and Sound-Alike (LASA) drugs. Cursive look-alikes (Plendil and Isordil) killed Ramon Vasquez. Sound-alikes plague phone-in prescribing by doctors. In 2003, the AHRQ published a list of medicines that amazingly look and sound alike both in their brand and generic names, and whose confusion has led to harmful errors.

Some of these pairings are terribly dangerous. For example, Adderall is a stimulant used to control Attention Deficit Hyperactivity Disorder (ADHD) that can raise blood pressure. Inderall, a beta blocker, lowers blood pressure and controls angina. No health-care provider wants a heart patient to swallow Adderall, which could be fatal. Likewise, Zyrtec is an antihistamine allergy medicine. Zyprexa is a powerful anti-schizophrenia drug that can cause brain and movement disorders, and diabetes.

All of these drugs should be prescribed with the utmost care. The FDA no longer approves new drug names that look or sound similar to existing medications. Perhaps more importantly, since 2001 the FDA has directed the use of "tall man" lettering on labels of drugs, whose similar names differ by syllable, in order to make sure the substances are not confused. You might see, for example, prescriptions for "celEBREX," an anti-inflammatory, and "celEXA," an antidepressant.

Since the late 1990s, the greatest strides against medication errors have been made through Computer Provider Order Entry (CPOE) systems now found in most large hospitals. Also known as e-prescribing systems, this ordering software screens for drug interactions, over and under doses, and adverse reactions with the patient's illnesses, allergies, lab values, and current medications. In hospital settings, CPOE has been shown to reduce medication errors up to 85 percent.

There are drawbacks. Excessive time at the computer can lead to reduced time at bedside which correlates with poor patient outcomes. Plus, some studies have shown increased medication errors during the early phases when CPOE is brought on stream. But, all things considered, there is no substitute for CPOE as a means of clear and consistent communication among physicians, pharmacy, nurses, and, above all, the patient, and for keeping the medications accurate during all stages of care.

Yet, an early order consistently passed through the system and among transcribers, pharmacists, nurses, and administered fully to the patient can still be a problem. The prescription can be flawed from the outset. Even if initially accurate, it can become ruinous if it is not reconciled to the patient's evolving lab results, progress, and vital signs at milestones called care transitions, and eventually at discharge.

Studies show initial orders tend to stay in the system throughout the care cycle, even if they are no longer needed or if they adversely interact with medicine a doctor subsequently orders. We do not know all the reasons for these lapses, but it seems that the deferential residents and nurses who provide most of the care are loath to countermand full-fledged attending physicians who sit atop the clinical totem pole.

Plus, those providers who should be conducting medication reconciliations often are hospitalists and residents who reach the ends of their shifts lacking the time to go into the computer to make the necessary deletions and dosage changes. They pass medication discrepancies along to their successors. According to an extensive review article in the *Annals of Internal Medicine*, "up to 67 percent of the patients admitted to the hospital have unintended medication discrepancies, and these discrepancies remain common at discharge."

The trouble can begin during or even before admission, unless the patient provides a Best Possible Medication History that covers all prescribed and not-prescribed medications. In the pre-computer era this process was known as a "brown bag review," since patients would dump their bottles, vials, and packets in front of a doctor or nurse who would record them and look up their interactions and side effects.

That still occurs today, but increasingly the clinician taps into the hospital's database as well as those of other treating physicians, and the patient reveals all his supplements, herbs, or other remedies. If he is on Medicare, Medicaid, or in the military, then the government's databases and formularies are accessed. Additional third parties should be contacted including family members, friends, caregivers, and doctors from the past whose prescriptions still may be getting swallowed.

In order to prevent adverse drug reactions, medication reconciliation, called "med rec," should take place at every care milestone such as when the patient moves into or out of the ICU, when lab values change, or when a drug no longer is necessary or working. Reconciliation shapes the patient's safety, and it identifies unintended discrepancies all the way to discharge, when the "best possible medication discharge plan" reconciles the discharge prescriptions from *all* physicians to assure that they harmonize.

So critical is medication reconciliation that it now is mandated by all health-care accreditation bodies in the United States and Canada, including the august Joint Commission. However, scrutiny occurs only during visits by accreditation teams. These agencies lack the budgets, police, investigators, or spies to monitor practitioners, pharmacists, and nurses on a day-to-day basis. Probably they should have bigger inspection staffs.

Pharmacists play a large role in the medication system—dispensing—but create a small proportion of errors (4 percent). In fact, we know that hospital pharmacists are practically flawless, when not overworked. One study showed that they usually make no errors if they don't have to fill more than twenty-five prescriptions per day.

Pharmacists do more than the mere mechanical acts of counting pills, putting them in vials, and handing them out. They consider the drug and dosage in light of the disease and the patient's various blood scores and levels. Pharmacists prevent errors by dispensing drugs in packets that require no mixing or dilution by nurses, and by walking the floors and rounding on patients as members of the "care team." These practitioners are known as clinical or decentralized pharmacists.

Published in *Pharmacotherapy* in 2001, the largest multi-center research study to date surveyed 430,586 medication errors at 1,116 hospitals. Hospitals using decentralized pharmacists posted a dramatic 45 percent decrease in medication errors compared with institutions that lacked these professionals. In regard to 17,338 reported errors that negatively impacted patient outcomes, including permanent injuries, death, increased lengths of stay, and additional drug therapies, the contrast was twice as stark: decentralized pharmacists yielded a whopping 94 percent decline versus centralized pharmacists. The authors, themselves academic pharmacists, correctly concluded "that one of the most effective ways to prevent or reduce medication errors is to decentralize pharmacists to patient care areas. The results of this study should help hospitals reduce the number of medication errors that occur each year."

Smaller studies echo the profound impact of clinical pharmacy. One led by Lucian Leape and published in *JAMA* focused on an intensive care unit, a department where nurses and physicians regularly reconcile medications in conjunction with constant rises and falls in patients' conditions. In a shifting scene of evolving labs, tests, scans, x-rays, and procedures, applying a clinical pharmacist to the care team cut medication errors by two-thirds.

Pharmacists often simply know more about drugs, families of drugs, and their minute gradations, than do doctors and nurses. A pharmacist at bedside performs an invaluable service when he hears a physician make a poor or erring order and stops it from entering the system and impairing care over the course of repeated shifts and probably until discharge.

Yet, a decentralized pharmacy is a luxury rarely found in American hospitals. A national shortage of pharmacists makes decentralized pharmacists expensive additions to staff, since these clinicians cannot bill for diagnoses or procedures. Conversely, simply billing prescriptions to insurers or Medicare for drugs dispensed from behind a counter keeps pharmacists off hospital floors. Like other safety priorities, this one takes a back seat to market forces, causing decentralized "strategies," according to Dr. Robert Wachter, an internist and patient safety expert at the University of California Medical Center in San Francisco, "to be relatively underemployed."

Unlike pharmacists who handle medicine constantly but cause few errors (and if re-deployed clinically would prevent many more), nurses follow ordering physicians as the second leading culprits in creating snafus. Thirty-four percent of medication errors happen during the administration phase of the process. In hospitals, clinics, and nursing homes, nurses pass out the pills, load the intravenous bags, hook up the lines, and insert the tubes that reach the system's end-users—its patients. Analysts generally count between ten and fifteen steps in the medication process, each of which provides an opportunity for error and harm. Nursing handles the last and most dangerous. Almost half of prescribing errors are intercepted before they reach the patients. But data shows that mistakes reaching the administration stage are halted only about 2 percent of the time. A chilling study of thirty-six health-care institutions showed that mistakes occurred in almost 20 percent of the doses administered and ingested.

Why? The simple answer is that nurses have a difficult lot. They receive wrong orders and push them. Drugs come in lookalike vials that are difficult to distinguish. Orders that come from multiple attending physicians can be unclear, even contradictory, and the doctors may be off-duty or hard to reach for clarification. Tubes and lines also look alike. When a patient returns from brain surgery with an intracranial drain, a nurse in haste might inject morphine into it instead of into the patient's central line. Or, a nurse who has a heart patient might crush Cardizem (a calcium channel blocker intended to reduce blood pressure) and pour it into the patient's nasogastric tube, crucially missing the "do not crush" order in the medical record for the timed-release drug. The patient will suddenly receive the full force of the drug, go into "asystole"—a cardiac stand-still without contractions—and die. Or, a resident who fails to perform his "sign-out"—inputting new medications or deleting unneeded ones at the end of his shift—causes a nurse to pro-ceed with an expired medication administration record. Or, a nurse mixing or diluting medications might become distracted by another call. Or, a nurse in possession of the correct med-ication in the right dosage could go into the wrong room and administer it to the wrong patient.

One in four Americans has received or has a family mem-ber who has received the wrong medicine from health-care pro-fessionals. Most were administered by nurses, who are trained according to the profession's "5 Rights" or "5 R's": right patient (using two identifiers, such as name and birthdate), right drug, right dosage, at the right time, and by the right route. Increas-ingly, four additional "R's" now are added to the list for drug administration including: right reason for the drug, right demon-stration, right to refuse the medication (by the patient), and right evaluation and monitoring.

In the main, nurses are dedicated, but they are in short supply, overworked, and forced to multitask to an absurd degree. Though some of the problems with drug administra-tion are beyond their control, many can be corrected upstream. For instance, the pharmacist can deliver medications in mea-sured packets to avoid mixing; residents also can be forced to use reconciliation software in their sign-outs. At times when nurses must handle, mix, or dilute medication, it can be done in designated quiet rooms that are free of distractions and hopefully include another nurse double-checking the procedure.

But a bigger breakthrough, and one borrowed from the digital inventory controls of other industries, involves bar coding. Beginning in 2004, the FDA mandated that all prescription medications, over-the-counter drugs, and biologicals, including flu, shingles, and pneumonia shots, but excluding blood products, carry bar codes. The FDA does not hold regulatory power over private providers like hospitals and clinics, but the government imposed bar coding on Department of Veterans Affairs hospitals, which became leaders in error and infection control. The results were impressive. In one landmark study at the vast VA Medical Center in Topeka, Kansas, bar coding dropped medication errors by 86 percent. Studies in non-government hospitals generally confirm a better than 50 percent reduction in medication errors with bar coding.

Resembling checkout scanning in supermarkets, this technology has become common in modern mid-size to large hospitals. The nurse must swipe three bar-coded items: the medicine vial, the patient's wristband, and the nurse's own badge, which ensures that this is the right clinician to administer the drug or drip, and stops someone else from doing it again later. If the patient is sentient and able, he can supply answers to basic identifiers like name and date of birth. The triple electronic match plus double human vocal checks make for a fairly safe system.

An even safer system called radio frequency identification (RFID) borrows from the passive tolling on highways, where a car with a billing device simply goes through a sensor. In RFID, medicines, patients, and nurses are microchipped. They produce alerts if the wrong pills, patients, or nurses enter a room.

However, bar-code medication administration (BCMA) seems to be beating RFID in the health-care information technology arena, probably because it costs less. BCMA can fail, especially when neonatal patients are too little to wear wristbands, or with elderly or burn patients whose skin is too frail to tolerate them. Triple-swiping has a bad reputation for being time-consuming and some nurses have created work-arounds, such as gathering the wristbands from all their patients and scanning them at one time in the hall. Other nurses do not like to scan and wake sleeping patients to give them drugs, so they put the bands on bureaus or trays and swipe them—or not.

Bar codes at a minimum are programmed to include the first two R's: right patient and right medicine, while some systems encompass the other three: right dose, right route, and right time. Some now even interface with the computerized physician order entry and the electronic medication administration record. More data can mean more potential discrepancies that lead to annoying buzzers, grim caution triangles, and skull-and-crossbones poison warnings on screens. Many discrepancies are insignificant and innocuous, and some providers suffering from "alarm fatigue" disable, work around, or ignore scanning, but they are in the minority. In the main, after reasonable training, scanning works to protect patients, prevent errors, and reassure nurses, whose routine increasingly involves a new aspect of patient empowerment. As patients are advised to tell providers not to touch them without washing their hands, in safer hospitals they are advised to refuse medication from a nurse who fails to scan them.

CHAPTER NINE: The Dream and Tragedy of Electronic Medical Records

The significance of Electronic Medical Records (EMR), sometimes called Electronic Health Records (EHR), does not stop with their profound safety net features in terms of catching errors. Rather, EMR is the great hope of the twenty-first century health-care profession, the long-awaited next step, regarded in the same way that transplants, cardiac drugs, antibiotics, polio vaccines, chemotherapy, and anti-AIDs drugs were welcomed in the twentieth century.

Put simply, the goal of EMR is to fuse instantly accessible electronic data with public health. It rests on two key promises: "interoperability" and a functional "universal clinical trial." Interoperability means that the computer at a patient's doctor's office can talk to the computers at his pharmacy, hospital, surgical suite, nursing home, dialysis clinic, dentist's office, phlebotomy iab, and to all the other archives of past and present medical records wherever he has lived, worked, traveled, and been medicated or treated.

The advantages of national interoperability are obviously huge. If an emergency physician in Indiana sees on his screen that his unconscious patient from Illinois has an allergy to penicillin, he won't prescribe it. If the electronic record shows one blood type, the doctor won't transfuse the patient with a different blood type.

The concept of the universal clinical trial is subtler but even more encouraging. Clinical trials test longitudinally (over time) how large groups of patients in different cities, countries, or hospitals cope with different drugs, diseases, and procedures. With universal medical records, a doctor treating a patient with a rare disease can probe the system to learn how other physicians around the world have fared with the problem. When treating a common disease like diabetes or hepatitis, and not getting good results with standard measures, a doctor can ask the system to find the records of similar patients around the globe who responded to something else, and obtain the information with anonymous search protocols that preserve patient anonymity.

Moreover, the data can be retrieved instantly in order to maximize the chance that someone may live or thrive with a different medicine or therapy. In some sense, getting help in this way is outside the box since it shortcuts the hidebound research, peer review, and publication cycle that takes years. But it also is in the best vein of one practitioner consulting other colleagues in order to solve a puzzle. Theoretically these consultants and their patients now can number in the millions.

The clamor for electronic records began in the early twenty-first century. Medical software companies sprouted like weeds. Suddenly there were about 1,700, some major, including installations of conglomerates like GE, Microsoft, and Siemens that hawked to a hungry but almost virginal market. The results were erratic, with doctors installing expensive systems, tearing them out, and buying others. At one point, the American Academy of Family Physicians advised its members to sit out the frenzy and stick with paper records.

There were costly system-wide crash failures. In my city, the venerable, highly-rated Children's Hospital of Pittsburgh installed a data system from Cerner Corporation, a unit of GE in 2002, with locked, passport-protected "closed source" code that required a doctor to make ten mouse clicks to issue a single order. In the emergency department now it took two doctors to care for a child—one to minister to the patient and another to ply a keyboard and screen. ER nurses no longer could grab medicines off a cart, but had to click through a digital dispensing labyrinth. In a famous study reported by the journal *Pediatrics*, a key metric—the mortality rate of children *in extremis* brought from other hospitals by ambulance to Children's for critical care—jumped from 2.8 percent to 6.6 percent after installation of the Cerner system.

In 2003, Cedars-Sinai Medical Center in Los Angeles installed a "state of the art" proprietary digital system for $34 million. Finding it cumbersome and time-burning, doctors rebelled, refused to use it, and it had to be torn down.

But there were successes too, including one in President George W. Bush's Texas hometown. In 2007, Midland Memorial Hospital, a 371-bed facility that had shuttled patient charts containing scribbled nursing notes from room to room and between floors in pneumatic tubes that tended to vanish, decided to go digital. Midland used "open source" software derived and customized from the famed and free Veterans Administration program called VistA, which is short for Veterans Health Information System and Technology Architecture.

The closed-source systems at Children's and Cedars no more could be modified than users of Microsoft Office could alter their Microsoft Word programs. At Midland the non-proprietary code could be accessed instantly by anyone in the system and modified and customized as necessary by authorized users. Key guidelines like anti-infection draping and antibiotic protocols came up on-screen for surgical patients. Infection rates plunged by 88 percent. Overall medical errors and deaths dropped. Because it was designed and adapted by medical professionals rather than imposed on them by business programmers, clinicians found VistA intuitive and easy to learn in about two hours. According to the hospital's director of information, it "became part of the culture. It would be impossible to remove it."

It is difficult to say precisely when the move to health-care IT began. But in the late 1960s and early 1970s, overworked health-care professionals unable to keep pace with the kludge of ever-mounting, uneven, unreliable, unreadable patient records began trying to adapt computing and software to their jobs and problems. As the *New England Journal of Medicine* recalled, "Early health IT offerings were cutting edge, but contemporary EHRs lag behind systems used in other fields."

One brilliantly creative system emerged in 1966 from a lab in Boston. According to the *NEJM*, the Massachusetts General Hospital Utility Multi-Programming System (MUMPS) "partitioned precious computer memory so parsimoniously that with only 16 kilobytes, the earliest personal computers could run an EHR supporting multiple users."

In an era not as fastidious as ours about intellectual property ownership and licensing, MUMPS "migrated" to other systems as they absorbed doctors and nurses from MGH. One, the Veterans Health Administration, known commonly as "The Vet," had a horrible national reputation for dirty, negligent, reckless, hazardous treatment that became a cruel joke on patients and the taxpayers and that was satirized in the 1992 movie *Article 99* starring Kiefer Sutherland. Today, with eight million patients, 180,000 employees, 163 hospitals, over 800 clinics, and 135 nursing homes, the Veterans Health Administration is the largest integrated health-care system in America. For over a decade it probably was one of the best.

One reason is VistA, and the people behind it known as the "hard hats." In the post-Vietnam era, when the system was crushed with disabled soldiers, the hard hats—an underground group of VHA doctors, nurses, and technicians—used MUMPS as a basis to create VistA and spread it into every function in the system, from patient care, to billing, to labs, to pharmacy, to dentistry, to medication prescribing, and beyond.

Sue Kinnick, a hard-hat nurse at the VA in Topeka, Kansas, went on vacation in 1992. Returning a rental car, she became inspired when the check-in agent simply passed a wand over the vehicle and her contract and printed a receipt. "If they can do this with cars," mused Kinnick, who glimpsed the future of error prevention, "we can do this with medicine."

Using hard-hat public domain code, Kinnick and other VA techies wrote scanner software. In Topeka, they gave patients and nurses wristbands, bar-coded medications, and passed out wands. Before administering meds, the nurses wanded the patients, themselves, and the pills. Since the system immediately stopped four problems—wrong patient, wrong drug, wrong dose, and wrong time—all VA facilities replicated it and preempted thousands of fatal dosing errors.

Fulfilling the great promise of digital medicine, VistA transformed the VA, a story reported in Phillip Longman's book, *The Best Care Anywhere: Why VA Health Care Is Better Than Yours*. The open-source program cut wait time for patients and drug dispensing errors. In one study, 5.7 million prescriptions were filled without a flaw. As efficiency rose, medical errors fell, and so amazingly did the costs per patient, which dropped a third by 2010, the same amount that they rose per capita in the private sector. Studies repeatedly showed that the VA provided Americans best levels in terms of patient safety and satisfaction as well as in the crucial quality indicators of the staff's frequency of following established clinical protocols.

Moreover, with VistA, VA physicians focused on broad-spectrum data mining that became the kind of large real-time clinical trial long sought by the profession. Applying VistA to the VA's millions of patients, researchers found a correlation between Vioxx (then a leading arthritis drug) and heart attacks that led to pulling the medicine from the market. Through sophisticated patient tracking, the VA substantially increased cancer and cholesterol screening as well as beta-blocker protection against heart attacks. It pumped up the pneumonia vaccinations rate from 29 to 94 percent, which epidemiologists showed saved 6,000 lives.[1]

Because of VistA's open source, non-licensed, un-copyrighted, non-proprietary nature, anyone could obtain a basic form of it under the Freedom of Information Act. The health systems of the Bureau of Indian Affairs and Department of Defense absorbed it, as did the public hospitals of Hawaii, West Virginia, and Colorado. In fact, over 85 nations have sent delegations to the VA to assess VistA and a host have used variants of it in their national electronic health data platforms, including Brazil, Germany, Finland, India, Jordan, Malaysia, and Nigeria.

Digitizing the American private health sector did not go as well. In 2009, a physician faced an average cost of $33,000 to install an electronic medical records system. For hospitals, it could climb to ten or even hundreds of millions of dollars. In a wasteful disaster, Sutter Health engaged industry leader EPIC, a Wisconsin software giant, to install EMR throughout the system's twenty-seven hospitals in Northern California. Begun in 2004, Sutter committed $154 million to the project's completion scheduled for 2006. Neither the costing nor timing proved accurate. By 2009, only one hospital was wired with EPIC, and the full system build-out would have required a billion more dollars. Claiming it could not fund both employee pensions and bear the burgeoning IT costs, Sutter stopped the project.

By 2009, less than 2 percent of private hospitals had fully integrated IT. Most obviously had some functions on computers—usually labs and billings. Physicians also had fragmentary office packages that they used in conjunction with paper files and prescription pads. Patchy IT led to errors. For instance, two phy-

---

1 As in other federal agencies, units of the VA health system have been plagued by understaffing, management problems, and cover-ups that have reduced the level of care. However, most of the significant gains made by the system remain in place despite the recent scandal.

sicians whose computers weren't communicating about the same patient might prescribe the same drug, leading to double-dosing. That year the Joint Commission warned that electronic records contributed to 25 percent of medical errors.

Wanting the electronic health record system to be safer and interoperable, the Obama administration set up financial carrots and sticks. Doctors would receive subsidies from Medicare up to $64,000 to make "meaningful use" of EHR. If they failed to convert to digital by 2015, their Medicare reimbursements would be cut. So far, more than $7 billion in federal funds dedicated to EHR have landed in physicians' offices.

But the starting gun went off and a real gold rush began in 2009 with the American Recovery and Reinvestment Act of 2009. The Obama Administration's $787 billion response to the financial crisis included $36.5 billion to create a national electronic medical records network. Hospitals clamored for hefty handouts of tax dollars to install or upgrade their digital architecture.

Passed with minimal public debate, the lucrative electronic subsidy was the handiwork of the Health Care Information and Management Systems Society (HIMSS), a registered lobby, and its "strategic partner," the Center for Information Technology Leadership (CITL), a non-profit. A powerful trade group, HIMSS represents about 350 industry leaders including GE Healthcare, McKesson, and EPIC. CITL publishes medical IT research that HIMSS distributes to Congress.

At the center of both groups and the chair of both boards was key Obama health-care advisor Blackford Middleton, M.D., a professor at Harvard and physician with Partners Health Care, the largest hospital system in Massachusetts. HIMSS pitched the bill based on CITL's estimates that full-scale electronic records conversion would save $77.8 billion annually, a figure that the watchdog Congressional Budget Office found "overly optimistic." But no matter: in his December 6, 2009 radio address, urging the legislation, President Obama claimed,

"We will make sure that every doctor's office and hospital in this country is using cutting-edge technology and electronic medical records so that we can cut red tape, prevent medical mistakes, and help save billions of dollars each year."

Middleton's research argued that the electronic savings could be realized only if the federal government stepped in with handouts. He professed not to be motivated by the financial gains that would be achieved by HIMSS corporate members, but only hoped to see medical care get better. "This is the nature of my dream," he told the *Washington Post*.

The stimulus money soon began to seem like the toy of special interests. The Department of Health and Human Services contracted with a non-profit group called the Certification Commission for Health Information Technology (CCHIT) created by HIMSS and headed by its former president, Mark Leavitt. In the increasingly murky world of high-tech money and acronyms, CCHIT performed the gatekeeping function of determining which IT products provided sufficient "meaningful use" to doctors and hospitals to merit subsidies. Although Leavitt took a leave of absence from HIMSS and continued to be paid by HIMSS while heading CCHIT, he insisted that he had no conflict, and that HIMSS member corporations held no edge over other EHR vendors. That raised eyebrows. As David Kibbe, M.D., an advisor on IT to the American Academy of Family Physicians put it: "One has to question whether or not a vendor-founded, funded, and driven organization should have the exclusive right to determine what will be bought by federal taxpayer dollars."

With its close ties to the Obama administration, HIMSS performed a great service to the for-profit proprietary sector of the industry when it lobbied Congress to exclude free-of-charge public IT programs and their offshoots from the mix for which doctors and hospitals would be eligible for stimulus money through CCHIT certification. That meant that open source VistA and its commercial non-profit variant World VistA would be kept out of health-care systems in favor of the products of the big boys who funded HIMSS, like GE, Siemens, EPIC, McKesson, and Microsoft.

But the real tragedy goes beyond fleecing taxpayers and clinicians. For one thing, about 60 percent of American physicians "rotated" through VA hospitals and clinics during their training and had used simple, intuitive, wiki-like VistA. Installing it in their practices, clinics, and hospitals would have vastly cut down on their learning curves (since they already knew a version of it) and decreased the drag on productivity and patient care from the buggy start-up with newly licensed IT, a period rife with medical errors and frustrations with managing data.

But why should "free" software be subsidized? Apart from the fact that it's better than the vast majority of its expensive licensed competitors—VistA won HIMSS' highest grade, a 7—the VA-derived program really is not free. It still requires substantial customization services and costs, which are far less than industry averages but nevertheless can run into the millions in a hospital and roughly $15,000 per doctor's office (a quarter of the available subsidy!).

Perhaps above all, the triumph of special-interest licensed products signals the end of interoperability and the long hoped for gains from electronic records. Dashing this dream also feeds into some of the worst behaviors of modern American health care—the tendency toward turf protection and maintenance of local monopolies that are costly, inefficient, and less than transparent.

Basically it works like this: local and regional health-care systems want to protect their market positions, especially if they're dominant. They resist sharing information—even vital patient data—with other providers. So if you are admitted unconscious or confused through the emergency room of one hospital, it probably won't be able to get your previous records from a rival system across town. Treatment will have to begin without your history of drug reactions, illnesses, allergies, and other conditions.

This situation was building before the Recovery Act and enshrined by its subsidies. Now hospitals pick and choose among hundreds of licensed closed-source proprietary programs that fund HIMSS and have been blessed by its cousin, CCHIT. These programs guard data, withhold it, and do not talk to each other. When physicians have the temerity to leave such a system and join a rival, they often face huge obstacles in transferring patient data even if the patients want to move with them.

In 2004, the Bush administration announced the goal that every American would have an electronic medical record by 2014, a goal that was not to be met though hundreds of IT firms crowded the field and pitched EMR to care providers. Since the technologies failed to talk to each other, the interoperability problem bloomed.

The Obama administration promised to expand the electronic medical infrastructure, leading to more communications, better treatment, and fewer errors. But instead of roads and bridges, the stimulus fostered a fractured world of feudal data kingdoms loathed by patient-oriented doctors, nurses, technicians, and administrators.

Marvin Malek, M.D., an internist and interoperability activist at Central Vermont Hospital, has written an article entitled "Health Information Technology is a Tower of Babel, by Intent." In addition to federal policy, he blames the Institute of Medicine, which recommended medical records as a way to stop medical errors. "But the Institute of Medicine . . . did not," he writes, "recommend the VA system's route towards computerization" which could use "a single popular software language to connect every hospital and doctor's office." Instead, "[i]n health care, we have created our own 'Babel' of incompatible medical software products. And this time, we can't blame God."

Psychiatrist and historian Carol Zisowitz's practice includes the severely mentally ill. Many of these patients have been involuntarily committed to treatment after numerous previous interactions with the medical and psychiatric systems from which she cannot readily retrieve records. This is dangerous and conducive to error because the gamut of psychotropic drugs she could prescribe is highly interactive with other medications that the patients could have "on board," and further could aggravate a host of physical conditions. Sometimes she is faced with the problem of having to prescribe with incomplete information.

A critic of federal EMR policy, she draws an analogy: "What if the government spent billions of dollars a year to build a phone system with which you could no longer call your next-door neighbor, much less your mother in California? Unfortunately, this is exactly what the Department of Health and Human Services is doing to encourage the use of electronic medical records. The need for health-care providers to communicate with one another is essential if EMRs are to save money and lives. Only by sharing information, with patient consent, of course, can they eliminate duplication of expensive services and tests such as MRIs, reduce exposure to radiation from unnecessary CT scans, and safeguard against prescribing medications which trigger allergies or hazardous interactions."

Zisowitz deplores the special-interest dominated Health Information Technology bureaucracy that flourished under the HHS Office of the National Coordinator (ONC), "which has a mandate to help providers select electronic medical records systems, [but] is not allowed, under provisions of the stimulus bill, to promote systems like VistA that are free of charge." ONC now has 62 regional extension centers that "are essentially websites with billboards for the largest vendors such as EPIC, Athena, and McKesson."

In November 2012, Zisowitz attended the annual meeting of the Academy of Psychosomatic Medicine, a discipline that recognizes the mind-body relationship in illness (contrary to the lay notion of imagined disease) and hence is especially important to mental health professionals. Ezekiel Emanuel, M.D., a prominent internist, oncologist, and bioethicist, then the special advisor to the Office of Management and the Budget, gave the plenary address. Like his younger brother Rahm Emanuel, President Obama's first chief of staff and currently Mayor of Chicago, Dr. Emanuel was no stranger to controversy. Sarah Palin and other conservatives falsely painted him as a proponent of "death panels" when in fact he opposed euthanasia. He carved out a strong if idiosyncratic position in favor of universal health care based on vouchers, blasted "single payer" insurance in deference to competition, lashed out at the waste in medical care, and proposed a ban on junk food.

In his speech at the 2012 conference, Emanuel extolled electronic medical records and the administration's policy. When Zisowitz challenged him and asked why the government did not simply advance VistA as an alternative to the clutter of private sources blocking interoperability, Emanuel's brief reply was that VistA support would amount to a government "monopoly" like "Ma Bell."

Emanuel may be a fine physician, but his point made little sense. In the 1980s, the break-up of the American telephone and telegraph ended the so-called Bell System of high-priced, consumer-unfriendly local monopolies. Washington's poorly thought-out policy of excluding VistA and its variants from the stimulus has reinforced and entrenched high-priced, dominant local "closed source" hospital systems that speak a babel of electronic record languages but not to each other and allow patients' risks of error inevitably to rise with the walls of information silence.

Another huge difference between the break-up of the Bells and the clutter of EMR platforms and providers is that subsequent sensible pro-consumer telecommunication laws forced the new telephone companies to talk to each other. That means that my Verizon cell phone can call your Sprint unit, and my Dell desktop can receive an email from your Apple iPad and so forth. Interconnectivity laws and regulations long have forced industry standardizations including in radio, television, trucking, and shipping.

But one must return to the mid-nineteenth century for an analogy to today's health care irrationality. Like hospital systems, railroads held regions in their iron grip and charged what they liked. They used a babel of narrow and wide gauge tracks to thwart interconnectivity and throttle competition. In the 1860s when the Lincoln administration and Congress promoted intercontinental rail service reaching to the Pacific, Washington imposed a standardized track width of four feet eight and one-half inches instead of perpetuating the feudal, Balkanized, price-gouging mess.

In 2008, without Bush administration support, Representative Pete Stark (D-CA) introduced a bill to create a low cost open-source electronic records highway under the auspices of the Department of Health and Human Services called the Health-e Information Technology Act of 2008. As Phillip Longman reported in the *Washington Monthly*, "HIMSS used its influence to smash the legislation." The following year, without Obama administration support, Senator Jay Rockefeller (D-WV) introduced the shorter but similar Health Information Technology (IT) Public Utility Act that died in committee without a floor vote.

Like single-payer health-care coverage, the notion of a nonprofit electronic medical records highway whether managed by the government or not probably is dead. Yet the dreams of an interoperable system offering comprehensive, user-friendly current medical, drug, treatment, and historical records for every patient as well as a vast national or even international clinical trial readily could become a reality.

In a system of carrots and sticks, providers already have been subsidized to install EMR while being told that their Medicare and Medicaid reimbursements will be cut if they are not on-stream by 2015. A small step that would cost Washington nothing but would save plenty of lives and tax dollars would be to warn hospitals and practitioners that they must become open-source by a certain date or else face financial sanctions from the Medicare colossus. "Providers," says Carol Zisowitz, "who wished to keep their proprietary systems could do so, but should eventually be penalized by government-funded insurance agencies if they refuse to make their EMRs nationally interoperable." The precedent already exists. As the babel breaks down, providers would become better informed and patients far safer.

CHAPTER TEN: Centuries of Hospital Infections

Of all the myriad hospital management problems, infection causes the most complications. Hospital-acquired infections (HAI) injure about 1.7 million patients and kill over 103,000 annually. Currently, between 5 and 10 percent of patients who enter hospitals for an acute illness or trauma pick up a "nosocomial" (facility-based) disease. The associated costs of these demoralizing, horrid, debilitating, and deadly bugs range between $30 and $40 billion per year.

While rare and shocking infectious agents like mad cow disease, swine flu, West Nile Virus, Ebola, and most recently, MERS (Middle Eastern Respiratory Syndrome) grab the news, four types of common scourges account for over 80 percent of hospital infections. Fortunately, we know a lot about them, including how to prevent them.

Urinary tract infections, often related to catheters, are the most frequent. They amount to about 35 to 45 percent of HAIs but result in the lowest costs and deaths. Surgical Site Infections (SSI) are second at 20 percent and the next lowest in costs. The last two types—Central Line–Associated Bloodstream Infections (CLABSI) and Ventilator-Associated Pneumonia (VAP)—each account for 15 percent of infections but are deadlier, costlier, and have been increasing rapidly.

For over a decade our society and government have been riveted by the problem of providing universal health insurance.

It is worth noting that about 18,000 die each year prematurely due to the lack of coverage. Over five times as many die from HAIs and the majority of them have insurance. However, we do not need to wait for the passage of landmark legislation, the outlays of hundreds of billions of tax dollars, or the creation of huge public and private bureaucracies, much less any form of scientific breakthrough, to quell this man-made epidemic. In fact, infection control ultimately results in net savings rather than costs.

Since the mid-nineteenth century it has been clear that poor hygiene, particularly hand hygiene, has been an unnecessary and preventable cause of death in hospitals. In the 1840s the Vienna General Hospital had the world's largest obstetrical program. It was divided into two wards. In Ward One, puerperal or childbed fever raged, killing 29 percent of mothers. In Ward Two, mortality peaked at 3 percent. The deadly disparity seized the attention of Ignaz Semmelweis, a newly graduated physician in his twenties who discovered a single difference in operations between the two wards. On deadlier Ward One, medical students assisted in childbirths. On safer Ward Two, mid-wifery pupils provided the care. So, Semmelweis conducted an experiment— he made the students switch wards. With the midwife students assisting on Ward One, the mortality rate plunged. With equal rapidity, it spiked on Ward Two now that medical students were working there. Still Semmelweis couldn't quite fathom the problem, although it seemed that somehow the medical students were communicating infection during childbirth while the midwives were not. Suddenly, Jakob Kolletschka, another doctor and forensic medicine professor at the hospital, died after cutting his finger during an autopsy.

Assigned to investigate the case, Semmelweis "found identical changes in [Kolletschka's] body and those of the childbed women." Now he knew what had infected and killed them: Unlike the training midwives, the medical students also dissected corpses and then appeared at childbirths with putrefied particles on their hands. In May 1847, a watershed moment in medicine and public health, Semmelweis ordered all staff and students involved in delivering babies to wash their hands first with chlorinated lime water. On both wards, puerperal fever rates dropped to around 1 percent.

Semmelweis' simple but brilliant experiment and lightning insight about iatrogenic infection fired the jealousy of the maternity department's supervising physician Johann Klein, who discharged Semmelweis in 1848. Obviously it would not be the last time that vanity trumped quality in health care. Fortunately, the following year, Semmelweis found a post in the obstetrics department in a Budapest hospital, implemented an antiseptic regimen, and brought mortality down to 0.85 percent. In 1861, he published the seminal *Die Aetiologie der Begriff und die Prophylaxis des Kindbettfiebers* (*The Cause, Concept, and Prophylaxis of Childbed Fevers*). Four years later, at forty-seven, Semmelweis, who had become mentally unstable and a patient at a Vienna psychiatric hospital, suffered a hand wound and tragically died of the same infection he discovered in the childbed women.

More than a century and half after Semmelweis' discovery, the U.S. Centers for Disease Control and Prevention found hospital hand hygiene in this country to be "abysmal," with reported compliance rates ranging from 5 percent to 81 percent. A 2010 review of diverse hospitals pegged the median at 40 percent. Amazingly, rates actually dipped more in ICUs where patients are more immunodeficient, sicker, and softer targets for infection. Overall, doctors were found to follow hand protocols less often than nurses. Long after Semmelweis, it seems incredible that the most basic and low-tech of infection controls remains spotty.

Moreover, hand hygiene is fundamental to all anti-bloodstream infection protocol "bundles," including those for central lines, urinary catheters, ventilators, and surgical incisions. It likewise figures into guidelines for preventing the spread of diarrheal germs like *Clostridium difficile* (*C. diff.*) and

drug-resistant organisms like Vancomycin-resistant *Entero-
coccus* (VRE), a streptococcus of the gut, and Methicillin-resistant *Staphylococcus Aureus* (MRSA).

Antibiotic resistant organisms constitute one of the tough-
est problems faced by modern medicine. Yet, an entirely doable
increase in hospital hand hygiene compliance from 60 to 80 percent alone has been shown to reduce them by 8 percent. Because
hand hygiene is so critical, it has been the subject of numerous scientific studies identifying blockers. Sometimes called
"system-level barriers," these include hurrying (usually due to
inadequate staffing levels), poor location choices for antiseptic
dispensers and sinks, weak or non-education on scrubbing and
gloving, and negative attitudes about the effects of antiseptics on
clinicians' own skins.

Since Semmelweis' survey of Viennese medical students
showed that some actually were washing their hands after autopsies yet still infecting and killing mothers, it has been known that
antiseptics generally work better than soap and water. Where
education fails, the false presumption persists of equality of hand
cleaning methods.

Soap and water still have their place; especially after touching bodily fluids and as a precaution against *C. diff.* contact. Visibly soiled hands must be washed with soap and water. In trauma
care and surgery, doctors and nurses who deal with grit, grime,
glass, and other foreign objects still must wash. Regardless, hand
hygiene cannot be perfunctory. Correct hand washing takes at
least fifteen seconds. With alcohol-based antiseptics, all surfaces
of the hands must be coated. A patient who sees less effort should
refuse to be touched by the offending clinician.

In the not too distant past, hospital infection control was
the province of epidemiologists and their staffs. A major socio-
cultural change has led to shared responsibility and "democrati-
zation," meaning equal rights to speak up against contamination
by all staff and patients.

So, how can we train clinicians to adhere to hand hygiene? One key concept involves "triggers," not to be confused with the electronic trigger tools used in calculating medical errors. Typical triggers compelling antisepsis or washing occur upon entering or leaving a patient room (even if the patient is not there) or before putting on or removing gloves when required, such as for insertion of central lines or catheters. Putting gloves on un-scrubbed hands is a waste—it simply leads to infected gloves.

Feedback in real time results in improved hygiene. A staff member is assigned to audit hand cleaning, essentially to monitor others on the unit. To keep the person from seeming like a spy or snitch, the part is rotated consistent with shared responsibility. Auditors give out "tickets" for non-adherent events. Copies go into employment files and can lead to discipline. To keep the audited environment from seeming too negative, positive tickets also are distributed for good compliance along with small amounts of money, meal rewards, and sometimes individually wrapped "Life Savers" candies. When the Acute Care for Elderly Medicine Unit, which served a vulnerable population at the University of Colorado Hospital, implemented real time punishments and rewards, hand hygiene adherence went up from 78 percent in January 2010 to 97.2 percent in June 2012.

Not choosing to enhance the culture of shared responsibility for infection control, some hospitals conceal the identities of hand washing monitors. Nurses particularly revile the spies who walk their floors, calling them "secret shoppers." Nor do the covert auditors seem especially accurate at tattling. For example, secret shoppers at Long Island's North Shore University Hospital claimed that 60 percent of providers scrubbed before going into a patient's room. When North Shore installed cameras, it found the actual rate was 6.5 percent. Moreover, real time videos raised the rate to over 90 percent, where it remained.

In hospitals, as at highway intersections, cameras serve as behavior management tools. Unfortunately, the hardware, software, and people to monitor the video feeds cost substantially more than adding an audit task—openly or clandestinely—to a nursing shift. Hence, cameras at washing stations remain rare. The Achilles' heel of patient safety is its low, weak, and unglamorous position when hospital boards pass a budget. But not to pay for infection prevention amounts to extreme short-sightedness and profligacy.

A decade ago, Allegheny General Hospital (AGH) in Pittsburgh studied the economic impact of infection on cases. The hospital should have made a profit on the pancreatitis treatment of a thirty-seven-year-old male. However, after the patient acquired the dreaded MRSA infection and stayed an additional eighty-six days, the hospital lost $41,813. A woman was admitted for routine stomach reduction. The surgery succeeded, but she endured a Central Line–Associated Bloodstream Infection (CLABSI), stayed forty-seven days, and an anticipated $5,900 profit turned into a $16,000 loss.

Between 2002 and 2005, AGH found it had 54 CLABSI cases in its coronary care and medical intensive care units. At that time, payments for CLABSI patients averaged $68,894 but the true costs of treatment were $91,733.50, so the hospital went into the red by $26,839 per capita and lost about $1.5 million overall. A broad study of Pennsylvania patients in 2005 showed that the average charge for patients who became infected almost quadrupled the economic outlay for patients who evaded this complication.

Parsing the problem further, a ten state study found that Surgical Site Infections (SSI) more than doubled costs at teaching (119 percent) and community hospitals (101 percent). Urinary tract infections jumped costs by 47 percent at teaching hospitals and 35 percent at community hospitals.

During the same period, the Institute of Health Care Improvement looked at Ventilator-Associated Pneumonia. It found that this common form of HAI caused per patient costs to rise by over $40,000. An analysis of MRSA at the University of Pittsburgh Medical Center showed that these infections added an additional $35,000 to the cost of each patient's care. In its important 2006 volume, *Unnecessary Deaths: The Human and Financial Costs of Hospital Infections* (2nd Edition), the Committee to Reduce Infection Deaths reported that in a 55-hospital survey an infection rate of only 4.09 percent was sufficient to erase inpatient profits.

Fortunately, as Peter Pronovost and his colleagues found, major HAIs can be eliminated provided hospitals commit to a cultural change plus provide resources that pale in comparison to the costs of infectious outbreaks. Before getting specific about the proven prophylactic protocols, two unifying, overarching themes must be mentioned. First, it bears repeating that hands must be cleaned before and after each patient contact. Second, active resistance, which exists everywhere, must be quelled for cultural transformation to occur. It can be done. But how?

According to a Joint Commission study, overcoming barriers requires data feedback comparing the hospital's rate of infection to regional and national levels. Choosing individual "champions" of effective methods makes sense provided that they have the respect of their peers among surgeons, anesthesiologists, nurses, and technicians, plus speak the language of the group they are guiding. Representatives of hospital management also must be brought into the mix and buy into the goals.

Undoubtedly the hardest task facing partisans of change according to the Joint Commission report involves coping with "organizational constipators," mid- to high-level leaders with clout who act as blockers and reactionaries. Efforts should be made to include or co-opt them and seek their "buy in." Failing that, try to "work around them." If unsuccessful: "Terminate the constipator's employment [and] take advantage of the turnover opportunities by hiring a person who has a very high likelihood of being successful."

Assuming acceptable politics and hand hygiene, the institution should implement "bundles," punch lists known to greatly limit SSI, VAP, CLABSI, catheter-associated urinary tract infection (CAUTI), MRSA, and *Clostridium difficile*. To minor degrees these bundles may vary across institutional, state, and national lines. But where instituted and obeyed, even in underdeveloped countries usually in accordance with World Health Organization protocols, they bring down infection rates dramatically.

The strategy to prevent SSI is well-evolved. It includes pre-hospital showering by the patient with antiseptic soap containing chlorhexidine, clipping rather than shaving the surgical site, a brief pre-operative stay, and "perioperative" antibiotics starting within an hour before surgery and stopping within twenty-four hours of incision closure. Aseptic conditions must prevail in the OR, including for staff attire, patient draping, and skin preparation. Since staff bring germs into the operating room, the number of people around the patient should be limited to those necessary. Surgical wound surveillance should be imposed to catch the signs of infection (redness, inflammation, pus) as early as possible. Post-operative "normothermia"—keeping the patient's temperature at normal with warmed IV fluids, hats, booties, and blankets—is a part of some bundles, since it helps with resistance to infection. Glucose monitoring to maintain blood sugar levels below 180 milligrams per deciliter fights infection as well as the onset of diabetes. If the glucose climbs too high, insulin is administered.

Among the most common HAIs, Surgical Site Infections historically show up in about one out of thirty "clean" cases. Infection rates rise in "dirty" trauma and emergency surgeries with debris. As surgeries lengthen, so does the chance for infection. Surgical patients with multiple illnesses ("comorbidities") also are at higher risk.

In dire straits, about 32 percent of patients on ventilators will die. Historically, about 15 percent will acquire VAP with a mortality rate (46 percent) that far outpaces other HAIs. To give intubated patients a fighting chance, VAP must be prevented. Workable strategic bundles focus on head-of-bed (HOB) eleva- tion of at least 30 percent that cuts the flow of gastrointestinal and upper respiratory tract matter into the lungs. Periodic aseptic suctioning also helps. As time on the ventilator lengthens, so does the likelihood of VAP. Strategies to wean off ventilators include daily stoppage of narcotics to "brighten" patients and get them talking, which is sometimes called the "sedation vacation." Fre- quent assessments by respiratory therapists geared to gauging the earliest moment when the endotracheal tube can be pulled out is vital. Peptic ulcer prevention with antibiotics can be ben- eficial, as is anti-thrombosis (clot) therapy that applies pressure devices to the legs. New studies also support using silver-coated endotracheal tubes that halt contaminated "biofilm" buildup, a cause of VAP. But hospitals have resisted purchasing these costly tubes, and they remain nonstandard. Finally, every clinician and person who visits a ventilated patient should have an up-to-date flu shot, wear disposable barrier protection garments, and prac- tice hand hygiene.

Repeated national and international trials have proved that the bundle approach pioneered by Peter Pronovost at Hopkins is effective against CLABSI that kills about 20,000 Americans per year. Central venous catheters should not be applied unless clinicians use barrier protections: sterile masks, caps, and gloves, as well as drapes to cloak the patient except at the insertion site, an area that should be sterilized with a 2 percent chlorhexidine gluconate solution. The femoral (groin) site should be avoided in favor of the subclavian artery at the base of the neck that supplies blood to the arms. As with ventilators, catheters must come out as soon as possible rather than be left to stay in and fester. So stop orders must be used and obeyed.

Lines should be changed after transfusions of blood and blood products. Transparent dressings or sterile gauzes must cover the insertion site and be changed whenever lines change. Catheters impregnated with antibiotic agents should be used with high-risk patients. The best practice, especially in the ICUs, calls for daily team meetings to discuss when the catheter can come out.

British sociologist Mary Dixon-Woods studied the interpersonal dynamics leading to the success of the Keystone Project in Michigan including over a hundred ICUs, and leading to the near eradication of CLABSI in all institutions regardless of size, wealth, teaching, or community hospital status. Dixon-Woods found a strong team ethic that "reframed catheter-associated bloodstream infections as a social problem and addressed it through a professional movement." The approach "harnessed data on infection rates as a disciplinary force." It used "hard edges" (i.e., the leaders were not afraid to be tough at times, using 'activist tactics and threatening sanctions against laggards when they were needed')."

So what should ICU patients, their families, and advocates do to prevent CLABSI? At minimum they should try to ascertain that the unit has a bundle or protocol in place and make sure that all clinical team members are dedicated to following it.

While not nearly as deadly as SSI, VAP, and CLABSI, Central Line–Associated Urinary Tract Infections (CAUTI) make up the biggest block of HAIs—about 40 percent. Indwelling Foley catheters are inserted into the bladder and serve as the point of entry for urine in a closed drainage system when it is critical for clinicians to know precisely the amount of liquid leaving the body in comparison with the quantity absorbed. When not handled aseptically or left too long in the patient, infection occurs. Other risk factors include age and malignancy.

In fact, catheterizations may not be wise. Resulting UTIs in young people can cause kidney scarring leading to renal failure later in life. So, parents should be satisfied that catheterization is a medical necessity before allowing it. Today, many men can qualify for "condom" catheters that cause less infection as well as pain and discomfort than inserted Foleys. Some studies also show that indwelling catheters treated with silver alloys or coated with microbial agents cause fewer infections.

All too often Foleys are used as management tools that reduce patient diapering, lifting, and bed panning. But when left in too long, these devices cause painful infections, lengthen hospital stays, and increase costs. Recently, like CLABSI and certain SSI, CAUTI appeared on Medicare's "No Pay for Errors List," a powerful tool to change clinician behaviors and prevent errors, the most prevalent of which is to forget that the tube is in the patient. A 2006 study showed that a third of doctors had no idea if their patients even had urinary catheters. The best practice seems to include automatic stop orders to remove them within two days. Patients and their families should be mindful about the necessity for urinary catheters, the continuing need for these devices, the existence of protocols for their sterile handling, as well as about the time they go in and the time that they must come out. If there is no stop order in the chart, they should ask for one.

Today, CLABSI, CAUTI, VAP, and SSI are seen as preventable HAIs. A common myth regards antibiotic resistant infections, especially MRSA and *C. diff.* as uncontrollable. The story of the growth of modern health-care contagion largely is the story of MRSA, which is among the most corrosive germs. Those who survive often suffer extensive hospital stays while undergoing repeated surgeries to excise infected tissue and sometimes bone. In 1995, MRSA accounted for about 2 percent of staph infections. Today it exceeds 60 percent. Hospitals stays for MRSA patients have climbed tenfold since 1995.

Other countries, including Denmark, Finland, and Holland, faced equivalent MRSA epidemics. After imposing rigorous screening and infection controls, they brought their MRSA to other staph ratios below 1 percent.

Studies show that MRSA contaminates about three quarters of patients' rooms. The vicious bacteria coats bed rails, tables, toilets, sinks, counters, curtains, and other surfaces. Whoever contacts it—patient, visitor, or clinician—becomes a disease "vector." Intriguing research revealed that nurses who entered a MRSA patient's room but did not touch the patient emerged 42 percent of the time with MRSA bacteria on their gloves. Clearly they must have touched *something* contaminated.

Another study found that doctors merely leaning over MRSA patients' beds resulted in their white coats being contaminated 65 percent of the time. This happens to be an easy fix: a clinician rounding on a MRSA patient can wear a one-time paper apron torn off a roll that is disposed of upon leaving the room.

A rugged bug, MRSA can live for hours on hospital surfaces and equipment. It seems to be more than twice as deadly as Methicillin-sensitive *Staphylococcus Aureus* (MSSA). Research on patients suffering bloodstream infections showed an 11.8 percent death rate for MRSA versus 5.1 percent for MSSA. Merely being in a MRSA breached environment or touching the bacteria is not enough to make someone sick. That requires the germ entering the body via a wound, lesion, incision, injection, drip, ventilator, or catheter. Very sick and old patients with open scars and intubation ports are particularly vulnerable.

Patients bring MRSA into hospitals. They leave its specks on wheelchairs, stethoscopes, floors under their beds, and the blood pressure cuffs that travel from room to room. In a 2006 study, 77 percent of mobile trolley cuffs contained MRSA contamination. A 2003 study showed that 63 percent of individual blood pressure cuffs and 53 percent of wall-mounted units bore contamination.

The period from 1976 to 2003 saw MRSA based HAIs multiply thirty-two times according to the Centers for Disease Control and Prevention. Moreover, about 70 to 90 percent of patients carrying the disease into hospitals were unknown to clinicians. In 1996, the *Journal of the American Medical Association* reported an "unprecedented crisis" due to antibiotic resistant infections.

In 2003, the Society for Healthcare Epidemiologists called for screening new patients for MRSA.

In fact, MRSA screening is simple. The inside of the nostril is swabbed, and then the product is cultured and conclusively analyzed within a day. It costs about twenty dollars, roughly the same as a fast HIV test. Researchers at Brigham and Women's Hospital using MRSA screens followed by patient contact controls and rigorous environmental antisepsis reported "profound" results, including a 75 percent ICU drop in MRSA. A Yale-affiliated hospital similarly saw screening reduce ICU MRSA infection by 67 percent. In 2006, the CDC recommended universal AIDS testing but controversially rejected "active surveillance" by nasal swabbing all patients for MRSA as too intrusive. Nevertheless about ten states now mandate MRSA screens during hospital admissions. The United Kingdom adopted screening for admissions to all "high risk" units. The British National Health Service MRSA bundle makes a great deal of sense:

1. Screen all patients admitted to "high risk" units, such as the ICU, cardiothoracic, orthopedic, and burn units.
2. Minimize movement of MRSA-positive patients.
3. Use gowns and disposable aprons when treating MRSA-positive patients.
4. Launder privacy curtains or use disposable curtains.
5. Decontaminate trolleys and wheelchairs after patient use.
6. Before surgery, attempt to decolonize MRSA-positive patients.
7. In the recovery area, segregate MRSA-positive patients.

As for the CDC, it seems to be relying on hand hygiene to quell MRSA pending more conclusive research on other methods, although over 50 studies have shown that precaution bundles including nasal screening, isolation, contact controls, and antisepsis following use by or on a MRSA-infected or "colonized" patient (meaning that the bacteria is present in the nose or on the skin) have reported effectiveness in reducing the spread of MRSA. On the contrary, studies have not shown significant reductions in MRSA "bacteremia" (the blood-borne infection of patients) from the hand hygiene education or from installing alcohol-based antiseptic dispensers outside patients' rooms.

A host of leading hospitals including Evanston Hospital (part of the NorthShore University Health System), New England Baptist in Boston, UPMC Presbyterian in Pittsburgh, and Veterans Medical Centers employ broad MRSA precaution such as screening of the "anterior vestibule of the nose."

The Society for Healthcare Epidemiologists (SHE) likewise recommends that "areas of skin breakdown" should also be sampled for MRSA. For a similar infection, Vancomycin-resistant *Enterococci* (VRE), SHE recommends rectal swabbing followed by equivalent antisepsis and precautions like "cohorting" VRE patients (keeping them together and isolated from the general population) and rigorous contact and cleaning controls. Patients should be "decolonized" of MRSA and VRE and other drug-resistant bugs to the extent possible with antibiotics and antisepsis. Unfortunately, once internal infection occurs, antibiotics that stop colonization may not work.

Clostridium difficile (*C. diff.*) causes infectious diarrhea in 1 percent of hospital patients, giving them a three times greater risk of death. The infection rate goes up with length of stay. Between three and four weeks, it rises by 13 percent. After four weeks, 50 percent of patients acquire it. Even hardier than MRSA, *C. diff.* spores last months on toilet seats, bed pans, urinals, rails, floors, call buttons, and television remotes. *C. diff.* exists in everyone's gut, but people taking chemotherapy or antibiotics have altered intestinal flora, permitting colonies to grow aggressively and emit high levels of toxins. Patients over 65 are at significantly greater risk.

Treatment bundles for *C. diff.* involve "enhanced" contact precautions. Basically, touching these patients should be avoided. Clinicians who come in contact must gown and glove before touching the patient, then remove and dispose of these items before leaving the room. After touching, hands must be washed with soap and water, a more effective measure against this germ than alcohol gels. Rigorous cleaning and complete disinfection of the room and equipment is necessary, especially before a new patient arrives.

Since the main indication for *C. diff.* is previous antibiotic use, "antibiotic stewardship" is required to decrease resistance to these drugs as well as infection. Narrowing the range of antibiotics should be explored as well as cutting them off when possible. Certain antimicrobial agents such as Clindamycin are known to stimulate *C. diff.* colonies in patients while others like Vancomycin and Metronidazole can be effective when used in bundles with barrier protections, sterilization, and hand hygiene as at Brigham and Women's Hospital, which reduced *C. diff.* by 40 percent. The hospital's "Contact Precautions Plus" may have played a role in this reduction:

CONTACT PRECAUTIONS PLUS

DISPATCH for room cleaning upon patient discharge/transfer

BEFORE entering	*BEFORE leaving*
1. Disinfect hands w. Purell (includes visitors)	Remove gloves
2. Put on gown (if having contact with patient or patient's environment)	Remove gown
3. Put on gloves	Wash hands w/ soap & water (includes visitors)

Infections can ruin and lengthen a patient's stay, expose him to additional surgery, damage, or kill him. So what can a patient, family, and advocates do to prevent this horribly discouraging, debilitating, and possibly deadly outcome? To the extent possible, the patient and allies should involve themselves knowledgeably with maximizing the positive effects of care and minimizing errors. The evidence-based strategies listed below can help patients stay safe and reduce vulnerability in a strange, complex, confusing, and dangerous environment:

1. If you are a surgical patient, ask the surgeon to give you chlorhexidine-based soap to shower with in the days before your admission.

2. Ask the surgeon or staff to provide you with his infection rate for the procedure in question. He should keep it and provide it. If it seems high, ask him to explain it, and if necessary and feasible, seek a second opinion.

3. Once in the hospital insist that everyone who touches you practices hand hygiene. That generally means scrubbing with alcohol-based gel from a wall dispenser, putting on gloves, touching you, discarding the gloves, and scrubbing again. If a clinician comes into the room gloved, ask if he washed after the last patient and before putting on the gloves and seeing you. If not, tell him to do it. Sometimes you cannot see the alcohol gel dispenser because it is outside the room or beyond your field of vision. If you ask if the doctor, nurse, or technician washed, hopefully they will tell you the truth. Not letting anyone touch you who has not practiced hand hygiene is your best chance for not picking up a communicable hospital disease.

4. For the same reasons, do not let a nurse or doctor press a stethoscope against your body that has not been freshly disinfected (rubbed with alcohol). The American Medical Association advocates that stethoscopes be cleaned for

each patient. Ask if this has been done for you. If you get a negative or equivocal response, insist that the clinician rub the device's diaphragm (the bell-shaped part) with alcohol in your presence. You also have the right to be assured that other pieces of equipment—blood pressure cuffs, wheelchairs, ear thermometers, and oximeters have been disinfected since the last patient and before they make contact with you.

5. From an anti-infection standpoint, any surgical or invasive procedure that is being done to you should require a protocol or "bundle" of safety measures. Ask to see it or have it explained to you whether it is for an incision, central line, insertion of a catheter, or intubation of a ventilator. If there is no bundle, that is not a good sign. If they will not or cannot give you the information, you can consider withholding your consent. If you need a central line, then request one that is treated to prevent infection such as with a silver chlorhexidine coating or impregnated with an antibiotic.

6. Ask for your own MRSA screening. A minority of clinicians and hospitals automatically provide it. In any event, you want it. Over a third of people have colonies of the germ in their nose, on their skin, or in existing wound sites. Screening is simple—a swift nasal swab will suffice. You want to be decolonized if possible before the material travels through an incision or intubation site into your body and seats there as a virulent infection. If you cannot be decolonized or clear the infection before the procedure, you want the clinicians and hospital to know about your status and take steps to prevent you from coming into contact with potentially vulnerable patients. If you are MRSA-free, you want the hospital and staff to take steps to prevent MRSA, *C. diff.* and other bugs from being communicated to you, and for them to reveal their prevention tactics in this regard.

7. You should stop smoking before surgery because smoking creates triple the risk of Surgical Site Infections and increases stay and recovery time.

8. You need to speak to your surgeon about limiting the size of the group in the operating room. More people have been shown to result in more infections.

9. You must object to having the surgical site shaved, which leads to tiny abrasions that become germ pathways. If clearing the site is necessary, then snipping or depilatories are preferred.

10. You need to be kept warm to resist infection better. It makes sense to request extra blankets, booties, a hat, and warmed IV fluids for your recovery period.

11. You want glucose monitoring, especially if you are a heart patient. While not especially well-understood, surgery raises glucose levels, which impedes the activity of infection-killing white cells in your blood. If glucose levels rise too high, you may need insulin therapy to control it, and you may need glucose monitoring even after discharge.

12. You want to avoid a urinary catheter if possible. If you are male and cannot avoid one, request a condom catheter. Also insist on a stop order and monitoring to ensure that a Foley catheter comes out as soon as possible. It is important to object to the use of catheters for incontinence management (especially in nursing homes) and for the convenience of nurses in understaffed units who lack time to toilet patients. Diapers and bed pans provide a better block to internal infection, but high levels of cleaning and infection must be maintained.

13. Remember that Caesarean sections are surgery. Mothers-to-be are becoming justifiably worried about infection. The risk of it is tenfold greater than from vaginal delivery. So it is important to establish that surgical checklists and full infection controls are in place before undergoing a C-section.

Perhaps above all you want to speak up, which is difficult when clinicians are both trying to treat you and rushing to do their jobs. But patients who speak up have better outcomes, and you do not want to complicate your illness, surgery, or treatment with an infection, especially if you can see the problem coming and speaking up could avoid it.

CHAPTER ELEVEN: Bedsores and Blood Clots

Some of the crippling and killing errors in hospitals and long-term facilities seem positively medieval. Indeed, they have been around forever in health care, though we know how to prevent or at least radically limit them.

The first, bedsores, also called decubitus (lying down) or pressure ulcers, cause about 60,000 deaths annually in the United States. About 2.5 million people will develop the painful and debilitating wounds each year including 5 percent of all hospital patients. Almost a third of spinal cord injury victims in community settings also suffer pressure ulcer complications. More than a million patients in acute care (hospitals) and long-term care (rehabilitation centers and nursing homes) develop these wounds. Despite the fact that they are largely preventable and that prevention is far simpler than the cure, bedsores are surging. Between 1995 and 2008 the Annals of Internal Medicine, which conducted a systematic review of studies, reported that they increased by 80 percent. The at-risk population of diabetic and elderly patients also is growing rapidly.

Bedsores erupt at a place where thin skin covers bony protuberances like the sacral/coccyx area of the lower spine, elbows, and heels. Especially in children, the trochanters (knobs at the top of the femurs) are likely sites that must be watched by caregivers and patients. Ulcers progress through four well-known stages:

Stage I: The skin is unbroken and intact, but signs of pressure such as redness, raised temperature, pain, or surface inconsistency emerge. At this moment it is vital for the patient to move out of bed, if possible, and call a nurse. It can take less than an hour for the sore to reach Stage II.

Stage II: Now a superficial open wound appears. Loss of skin occurs in the epidermis (top non-vascular level), or below in the dermis sometimes called the "true skin." An open or closed pinkish blister pops up, but there is no "slough" yet, meaning no dead tissue. Since failing to discover and promptly treat bedsores at this stage constitutes grave and inexcusable medical error leading to increased morbidity, mortality, and length of stays, the U.S. Centers for Medicare and Medicaid Services since 2005 has refused to allow payments for patients who suffer Stage III and IV ulcers.

Stage III: "Full thickness" skin loss occurs causing fat to be visible, but not generally bone, muscle, or tendons. Slough can be a factor.

Stage IV: Reflects extensive destruction of muscle, bone, or other supporting structures. There is slough and "eschar," sometimes called a "black wound" scab, made out of dead tissue and seen in burns and gangrene. The patient now is very sick, probably infected, and may die from something secondary to the condition that he sought care for in the first place.

∎

Realizing that prevention is key, in 1987 two Nebraska nurses, Barbara Braden and Nancy Bergstrom, developed the Braden Scale for predicting pressure sore risk. The scale scores six criteria: sensory perception, moisture, activity, mobility, nutrition, and friction and shear. The first five are scored from 1 to 4 with 1 signifying the highest risk. Friction and shear are scored from 1 to 3. The maximum (best) score is 23 and the minimum (worst) is 6. Points predict patient risk: very high (9 or less), high (10–12), moderate (13–14), mid (15–18), and none (19–23).

The Braden Scale has won near universal acceptance in health care. Probably all in-patients or their advocates should ask to be scored for their total points, and even for their internal scores in each of the six categories:

1. *Sensory Perception* means the patient's ability to sense pain or discomfort. If they cannot feel it, they cannot complain and thus must depend totally on providers and advocates to perceive sores at the earlier moment.

2. *Moisture.* When wetness through incontinence, spills, washing, or perspiration persist, skin "macerates," meaning that it thins, softens, separates, and withers. So moisture has to be monitored and dried immediately.

3. *Activity* matters because without it muscle atrophies and tissue erodes. To the extent possible, it makes sense to keep patients active: walking, washing, feeding themselves, toileting, and participating in physical therapy and other forms of movement. Of course, for the very ill, post-surgery patients, and trauma victims, not much activity may be feasible. But to the degree possible, patients and their advocates should ask for activity.

4. *Mobility* is the critical minimal litmus of activity. Scoring this means assessing whether patients have the physical capacity or will simply need to adjust their body positions in bed.

5. *Nutrition* is a key to health and strength of skin, muscles, and organs. The amount of food, adequacy of hydration, methods of ingestion (orally or by line), and whether patients can tolerate supplements need to be evaluated.

6. *Friction and Shear.* Friction comes from sliding in and out of beds and chairs. A term adopted from engineering, "shear" occurs when skin moves in one direction and bone in another causing capillaries and cell walls to break down.

Not entirely impressionistic, these categories contain objective measurements that made the scale provider-friendly (if they will only use it!). A Braden score sheet for predicting bedsores can be found online at www.bradenscale.com/images/bradenscale.pdf.

In order to prevent sores, patients must be scored upon admission. Radical changes in any or all of these categories are likely to occur with sedation, surgery, and until sickness ceases to progress. Hence, the Braden test should be repeated every day of hospitalization in order to stop ulcers or keep early stage wounds from becoming severe.

When patients score 12 or higher, the risk is high enough that they should be treated with a prophylactic protocol or bundle that at minimum includes turning or repositioning them at least every two hours. Typical bundles also include daily overall inspection of the skin. often with emphasis on vulnerable parts like the sacrum, buttocks, and heels, rigorous attention to preventing wetness, moisturizing dry skin, upgrading nutrition, and exercising. Even the sentient bed-bound may be able to participate in "range of motion" efforts. Others should be active to the extent possible and at least get in and out of bed. Types of beds and bedding are significant. For risky patients, foam beats standard mattresses as do low-pressure mattresses, sheepskin overlays, and high-tech beds that redistribute pressure.

Above all, the patient must be turned with less than two-hour frequency. But how do we get busy, overworked, distracted nurses to do it? One method seems to involve putting turning as well as exercise and inspection times on patients' in-room "care boards." But nurses have to go into the room to see this data and sometimes, due to lights off, under-staffing or other problems on the floor, they may not enter or see it in time to stop a wound. An array of devices on the patient's door seems to work, including ones that indicate the time until the next turning, and cut down on long lapses. One that staff likes and understands includes an imitation traffic light that is green during the first half of the period, yellow during the second, and turns red when time is up.

It is not going out on a limb to say that bedsores are regarded as preventable by most nurses but not by a lot of doctors. The notion that nothing has been shown to reduce them even pops up in some instructional literature for physicians. In 2013, the *Annals of Internal Medicine* published "Preventing In-Facility Pressure Ulcers as a Patient Safety Strategy" with financial support from AHRQ. Reviewing studies contained in principal databases such as MEDLINE and EMBASE, the authors found evidence that supported the positive effect of patient care bundles including two-hour turning and specialized bedding.

In addition, coordinated approaches to prevention called S.O.S. ("Save Our Skin") inter-disciplinary teams with dedicated leaders sometimes called "Skin Champions" who have the ability to educate and discipline worked well, as did posting records of how one unit fared against another in preventing ulcers. Some training exercises included attempts to modify behavior and have providers recognize the urgency of the problem. In one, team members sat on bed pans for half an hour in order to sensitize them to the fact that an ulcer can materialize that quickly. The *Annals* also reported studies showing real cost savings usually in the range of about a thousand to three thousand dollars per ulcer prevented. In 2008 a two-hospital system in Naples, Florida reported an $11.5 million savings from a documented drop in prevalence of ulcers through prevention.

About one out of forty bedsores leads to death. When ulcers do materialize they must be attacked aggressively with care strategies including debridement (removal of debris), and keeping surrounding skin dry while keeping the wound bed moist but free of "exudate" (pus) by using irrigation cleaning. Now normal saline generally is preferred over antiseptics. Sometimes electric currents are applied to ulcers. Regardless, bedsores involve deep tissue damage and serve as portals to local and systemic infection; so, it is always better to prevent them.

What can patients (and their advocates) do to prevent these errors and complications?

1. Ask to be evaluated preferably according to the Braden scale for the risk of bedsores. Know the score at care milestones and especially when mobility is limited or changes.
2. If found to be at risk, ask for low-pressure bedding and regular repositioning ("turning").
3. Insist on being maintained in the cleanest and driest possible manner.
4. Try to remain active and mobile even if bed-bound.
5. Immediately report any redness, pain, or pressure from lying or sitting.

Ask if the hospital has a bundle or protocol to prevent bedsores. It should. Ask to see it or for it to be described, know what it contains (e.g., turning every two hours and a daily skin inspection) and ask for a commitment that it be followed.

■

The Medicare Do Not Pay List also includes two types of blood clots that occur in hospitals: deep venous thrombosis (DVT) and pulmonary embolism (PE).

Forming a blood clot or "thrombus" in the vascular system during a hemorrhage amounts to a life-saving event. Otherwise, clotting constitutes a hazard since it clogs vessels and chokes off the blood supply to organs. When a thrombus detaches from its site on the vessel wall, it becomes an "embolus" that can cause a blockage at a distant point. A clot that travels from the lower leg to the lungs it is called a pulmonary embolus (PE).

While most pulmonary emboli resolve without harming people, in about 10 percent of cases "infarction" (death of lung tissue) occurs that can be fatal either through respiratory failure or a heart attack. Sometimes there are symptoms, especially "dyspnea" (air hunger and labored breathing) but often emboli go unnoticed. Regardless, autopsy studies show that about half of those who die in hospitals had a pulmonary embolism. Overall, PE is fatal to about 20 out of 1,000 sufferers.

Once PE is diagnosed, medical intervention can be tried with anti-coagulant drugs like heparin. If the patient cannot tolerate the resulting bleeding or is in critical condition—advanced PE can kill within two hours—then an emergency surgery called a "pulmonary embolectomy" should be attempted. Obviously, no provider or patient wants to reach this point.

Each patient and his advocates must ask to be evaluated for clot risk and receive a preventive strategy. For something fairly low-risk like an orthoscopic knee repair, the plan may be limited to "aggressive ambulation." For hip fracture surgery, low-molecular-weight heparin (LMWH) or a related synthetic anti-coagulant called fondaparinux begun before the procedure and continued afterwards with compression devices reduces risk substantially.

Surgery comes with an increased risk of thromboembolism. However, well-recognized and studied forms of "prophylaxis" (prevention) exist for most procedures. For low-risk surgeries, reported rates of DVT and PE are 0.4 percent and 0.2 percent respectively. For relatively high-risk procedures they climb to 10 to 30 percent (DVT) and 4 to 10 percent (PE). Other strategies can include walking, blood-thinning drugs, and tools such as pressure stockings and sequential compression devices that mechanically apply intermittent force to the leg and prevent 50 to 80 percent of clots. The medications, devices, and other therapies are chosen according to bundles that focus on patient risk factors, including obesity, age, sex, chronic venous stasis (congestion of the blood), reduced mobility, catheter insertion, and pregnancy.

Trauma adds risk, especially from fractures to the lower legs, thighs, and pelvis. Some high-risk surgeries for clotting include orthopedic, intracranial, gastric bypass, bowel resection, and kidney transplants, to name a few. Some of the diseases that make clots likelier are cancer, heart failure, lupus, chronic obstructive pulmonary disease (COPD), blood disorders, stroke, and inflammatory bowel disease.

In addition to movement, pressure devices and warfarin (Coumadin), the provider's arsenal includes undifferentiated heparin (UH) and low-molecular-weight heparin (LMHW) a refined, more powerful strain of the drug.

More challenging than preventing bedsores, anti-clotting prophylaxis involves meticulous medical intervention and serious potential side effects—bleeding—that itself can require emergency therapies including transfusions.

In 2012, the American College of Chest Physicians—the key doctor's association dealing with clots—called upon "every hospital to develop a formal strategy that addresses the prevention of VTE (venous thromboemboli). The adoption of such a course has been shown to reduce DVT and PE by over 40 percent. The medical profession knows that these strategies work. No one should enter a hospital that does not evaluate for clots, and treat prophylactically before, during, and after a procedure, including when the patient goes home.

Afterwards, by the way, can mean for four to five weeks. Discharge directions with an arranged hand-off to home treatment are critical. The ball must not be dropped here. The patient, if able, can be taught to give himself subcutaneous injections of blood thinners into the skin above the abdomen. If that cannot be done, the task must be transitioned to a caregiver or visiting nurse. Otherwise, a clot could ruin the recovery. Thus, providers, patients, and their advocates must be rigorous about this hand-off to stepped-down care, or else a fatal error could occur outside the hospital that has been caused by it.

CHAPTER TWELVE: Delirium and Falls

Lay people tend to see delirium as a rare kind of madness that mounts suddenly and often without cause, although it sometimes is popularly associated with anguish, trauma, and drug withdrawal. Medical professionals, especially in acute care facilities (hospitals) and long-term care (nursing homes), see a lot of delirium and consider it one of the worst complications of health care.

Like Libby Zion, patients with delirium tend to become agitated, unresponsive, and deeply confused. Obviously they cannot participate in care decisions, describe symptoms, report their medications, give a history, or follow directions. Like Libby they try to tear out their tubes. Like her they endure restraints and powerful antipsychotic medications such as Haloperidol which themselves sometimes lead to complications, injuries, loss of mobility, and further mental status changes. Like Libby, they sometimes die. In fact the 5 to 9 percent mortality rate associated with institutional delirium approximates that of sepsis (bloodborne infection) and myocardial infarction (a blood clot causing death of heart muscle tissue).

When not fatal, delirium often results in nursing home placement and/or the long-term loss of ability to care for oneself. Some clinicians anecdotally regard an episode of delirium in the elderly as a precursor to full-on Alzheimer's disease within a year or two though that has not been proven. About 10 to 30 percent of medical and surgical patients 65 and over will show signs of delirium. Approximately 80 percent of those in the ICU will have an episode; hence delirium sometimes is wrongly called "ICU psychosis."

A Mayo Clinic manual defines delirium as "an acute confusional state." Delirium sometimes is mistakenly lumped with dementia, but as Mayo puts it: "The primary distinguishing feature between delirium and dementia is the retention of stability of alertness in dementia."

Some patients present with delirium—about 40 percent of severe burn victims do. But more often, the disturbing and destructive behavior appears during treatment.

Also associated with post-operative complications, delirium results in longer hospital and ICU stays. Daily costs for delirium patients are more than double those of patients who do not manifest it. The national annual burden from delirium reportedly ranges from $38 billion to 152 billion, which does not include costs in post-acute institutions like nursing homes.

Studies show that about 10 to 20 percent of patients, mainly elderly, will be admitted to acute care facilities with signs of delirium, secondary to their reasons for seeking care. Astonishingly, about 30 percent, again mainly 65 and over, develop delirium during treatment.

∎

In the late twentieth century, practitioners at a host of hospitals, particularly Yale University, the University of Chicago, and the Cleveland University Hospitals stopped accepting that delirium was a common negative outcome that would mar care, and began developing patient safety strategies to prevent it.

Researchers have described delirium as "multifactorial," meaning that vulnerable patients usually have a gamut of risk factors: these include severe illness, dehydration, taking multiple medications, blood transfusions, comorbidities (such as diabetes in addition to the acute problem), catheterization, atrial fibrillation, pneumonia, alcohol or substance abuse, prescription neuropsychiatric drugs, low blood oxygen, fever, and being scheduled for certain procedures such as hip or heart surgery, as well as mental status changes like early signs of dementia, vision and hearing loss, malnutrition, sleep issues, chronic pain, constipation, urinary infection, and reduced mobility.

This knowledge is useful. Many of these problems can be addressed aggressively, hence delirium theoretically can be fended off before it materializes. Because delirium is a major insult to patients (from which they never may recover) and an impediment to care, better hospitals began implementing prevention programs. These prophylactic bundles, which focused on at-risk patients, often became known as Hospital Elder Life Programs (HELP). Studies show that where implemented they significantly reduce, but do not totally eliminate, attacks of delirium.

Probably the largest and best study occurred at Yale in the 1990s and led to a landmark 1999 article in the *New England Journal of Medicine* entitled "A Multi-Component Intervention to Prevent Delirium in Hospitalized Older Patients." Funded by the National Institute of Aging, a unit of the National Institutes of Health in Bethesda, Maryland, the study followed 852 patients age 70 and above who had at least one of four risk factors in a "predictive model" for delirium: visual impairment, severe illness, cognitive impairment, and a high ratio of blood urea nitrogen (an indicator of kidney function) to creatinine (a crystalline by-product of metabolism). The standard blood test for this ratio far more reliably shows dehydration than crude analyses like the weighing of fluid "ins and outs" that was provided to Josie King, who suffered from delirium and then died.

The Yale patients were divided into two equal groups. The first received the "usual care." The second, known as the "intervention group," received measures in six categories to prevent delirium: cognitive impairment, sleep deprivation, immobility, visual impairment, hearing impairment, and dehydration. These six were chosen because they were amenable to repair. Moreover, the fixes were low-tech, commonsensical, easily trainable, and readily measurable.

Cognitive impairment was quantified daily with a thirty-question test called the Folstein Mini-Mental State Examination (MMSE). It measures such things as "orientation" (date, season, name of hospital, floor, city, state, and country), "registration" (memory of three items one minute after they are mentioned), "attention and calculation" (asking the patient to count backwards by 7 from 100, and spell words backwards).

It is assumed that the elderly patient may have some cognitive difficulties, especially in a strange medical environment. Therefore, staff followed an orientation protocol including using a whiteboard with the patient's schedule, names of his care team, regular reminders of his physical location (room, floor, etc.), and thrice daily "therapeutic activities" comprised of discussions of current events, cards, word games, and recollections of family history. The goal, often achievable, is to raise the score on the orientation portion of the MMSE.

Each day patients also had sleep deprivation assessed. Interventions included soothing non-drug bedtimes with warm milk or herb tea, back massage, and relaxation tapes or music. Noise from pagers, call buttons, medical machines, hallways, and staff was suppressed as much as possible. Planned sleep interruptions for medications, vital signs, x-rays, and procedures were re-scheduled. The goal was to maximize sleep and minimize or eliminate sedative use.

The next delirium risk factor was immobility. The intervention included "early mobilization": getting the patient to walk as soon as possible, or if not possible, to perform range of motion exercises while lying or sitting. Mobilization also meant eliminating or limiting "binders" like restraints and catheters. Success with this intervention was recorded by gains in the

Katz Index of Activities of Daily Living, which assesses feeding, continence, transferring (from bed to chair), toileting, dressing, and bathing, and assigns one point for success in each of the seven core functions.

The fourth risk factor was visual impairment. Patients experiencing it were supplied with glasses or magnifiers, large lighted telephone keyboards, and glowing call bells. The goal was correction of visual difficulty within the first two days.

Fifth, hearing impairment, was measured by the "Whisper Test." From three feet behind the patient, a staff member whispered twelve times. If the patient heard less than six whispers, he received interventions including portable amplification devices and impacted ear-wax removal with the goal of improving the number of whispers perceived on daily tests.

Finally, dehydration was assessed according to the blood urea nitrogen to creatinine ratio. Since the normal range was between 8 to 18 (both in milligrams to deciliters), above eighteen signified the need for the additional drinking of liquids until the ratio descends to normal.

The Yale study ended with the application of a universally accepted algorithm for determining delirium both to the usual patient group and the intervention group. Called the Confusion Assessment Method (CAM), it has four stages: (1) "acute onset with fluctuating course"; (2) "inattention" (the patient loses focus and the ability to follow a conversation); and either (3) "disorganized thinking" (incoherent or irrelevant speech); or (4) "altered consciousness" (either the patient is hypervigilant and hyperactive or lethargic and hypoactive).

The CAM showed delirium in 15 percent of the usual care group versus 9.9 percent in the intervention patients. The difference in occurrence of more than 50 percent was significant. In fact, prevention should have been even higher since researchers recorded "non-adherence" by interventionist staff that varied according to protocol. For instance, 92 percent adhered to the vision protocol. But adherence dropped to 81 percent for increased fluid intake, and strangely plunged to 71 percent for the non-pharmacological sleep measures. So the overall intervention success rate could have been even better.

In 2013, the *Annals of Internal Medicine* with support from the Agency for Healthcare Research and Quality analyzed nineteen studies and reported that "most multicomponent interventions are effective in presenting onset of delirium in at-risk patients." The *Annals* also listed "The Most Common Components of Successful Delirium Prevention Programs":

Anesthesia protocols
Assessment of bowel/bladder functions
Early mobilization
Extra nutrition
Geriatric consultation
Medication review
Pain management
Prevention and treatment of medical complications
Sleep enhancement
Staff education
Supplemental oxygen
Therapeutic cognitive activities/orientation
Vision and hearing protocols

Like infections, bedsores, and blood clots, delirium no longer can be tolerated as an expected treatment outcome. Not to prevent it, or at least try to prevent it, is a grievous structural error in care.

What can patients do? Certainly they or their advocates should ask for screening to determine if the patient is at-risk (most elderly will be) for developing delirium. They should seek prevention protocols, which might be called HELP programs or something similar. It also makes sense for anyone at-risk to have a familiar companion. Hospital rooms can be visited by 20 to 40 strangers per day—doctors, nurses, residents, technicians, cleaners, clergy, dietary staff, social workers, and insurance checkers to name a few. Some clinicians believe that this unfamiliar parade kindles paranoia in confined, debilitated people that can kick over into delirium (we do not really know the mechanism of delirium, but many metabolic or emotional changes can trigger it). For some, an antidote can be a familiar person, who allays fear, answers questions, dispenses doses of reality, and provides connections to the patient's normal and healthier world.

Like delirium, falls are a particular bane of the elderly, considering that 30 to 40 percent fall each year, and 10 to 15 percent endure fractures. About half the patients in long-term care fall annually. One in five institutionalized patient falls leads to a serious injury such as a fracture or head injury. Not surprisingly, the "fear of falling" in older hospital patients outpaces worries about being misdiagnosed or given the wrong test or procedure. Falls produce increased lengths of stay by an average of seven days with added costs of about $14,000. The idea of a fall seems clear enough, but the medical profession has difficulty defining one. The National Data Bank of Nursing Quality Indicators defines a fall as "an unplanned descent to the floor with or without injury." To the World Health Organization, a fall is "an event which results in a person coming to rest inadvertently on the ground or floor or some lower level."

Probably every patient should be assessed for risk. With age come changes that lead to falls, particularly in cognition, vision, and the onset of comorbid diseases like Parkinson's that impact motor skills. Among the best predictors of future falls is a fall that has occurred in the past year.

Outside of the hospital, the elderly should be screened for falls, which at minimum means asking their history of falls and identifying risk factors such as balance difficulties, arthritis, psychotropic medications, problems with proprioception (overall coordination: hand-to-eye and body in relation to physical objects), and muscle weakness.

Clinicians in ambulatory practices may not have many chances to stop blood clots or bedsores, but they have plenty of opportunities to prevent falls. About 30 percent of seniors in the community will fall each year with the rate rising to 50 percent among octogenarians.

Falls constitute a public health problem, not just in this country but worldwide. Particularly prevalent—there are about 340,000 annually in the U.S.—hip fractures combine two grave issues: diminishing bone material and the increasing propensity to fall. After age forty, both sexes endure bone loss of about 1 percent per year. However with menopause the rate in women jumps approximately 3 percent annually for about seven years and then returns to the normal single percent loss. As a result, women have about twice the rate of broken hips and wrists, plus eight times the rate of spinal compression fractures, when compared to men.

Two main forms of bone disease that plague the elderly often exist simultaneously and can be limited, thus staving off falls. In osteoporosis, the bones lose both mineral and non-mineral tissue. Porosity increases when the Haversian Canals (the fine channels in bone that transmit nutrients) widen. It is a common misconception to think of all age-related bone loss as osteoporosis for which there is no cure; the condition can be slowed by supplemental estrogen, which is no longer recommended, or calcitonin, a thyroid hormone. Osteoporosis constitutes most but not all bone weakening and loss in the elderly.

Other older patients have osteomalacia ("bone softening"), a strictly mineralized loss. Both preventable and treatable, osteomalacia results from a lack of vitamin D faced by many housebound or institutionalized older people that is aggravated by reduced abilities of the skin and gut to make and absorb the vitamin.

Interestingly, there is a spike in hip fractures in late winter and early spring that cannot be accounted for by bad weather–related accidents. Twice-a-week sun exposure for about fifteen minutes can treat osteomalacia, with perhaps more exposure recommended for darker-skinned people. Regardless of skin color or race, seniors probably should take 800 international units of vitamin D daily in diet or pills, plus 1,500 milligrams of calcium either in supplements or food, which may reduce the risk of fracture. It also makes sense to limit other pharmacological causes of bone loss like corticosteroids and heparin when possible as well as excess alcohol.

Hip fractures are dreadful problems. About 20 percent of elderly patients who suffer them will cease to thrive and die within a year. Almost all occur in the course of falls, though a few happen through torsion of severely osteopenic (depleted bone tissue) femurs. Surgery has to happen fast—within 24 to 48 hours. After that amount of time, morbidity and mortality rise rapidly as do complications from pneumonia, blood clots, bedsores, urinary tract infections, and delirium.

About a fifth of elderly hip-fracture survivors end up in nursing homes because they no longer can walk or care for themselves. More common than hip fractures and usually not caused by trauma, osteoporotic vertebral fractures lead to major loss of height and spinal curvatures that used to be called "dowager's humps." Like hip fractures this is largely a female condition. Chronic spinal pain from it can be severe. In 2004, the U.S. Surgeon General published a report on osteoporosis that revealed that 1.5 million people experience a fracture annually and that the costs of care were $18 billion.

Among the most important things community health-care providers can do for elderly patients is to help them avoid falling. As in so many areas, prevention begins with evaluation, which, as with delirium, calls for a multi-factorial assessment. It is not ironic that the clinical treatment that patients receive is known in the medical profession as "ambulatory care." It has no more critical mission than to keep people as mobile as possible and to prevent threats to mobility from falls and fractures.

The evaluation starts with a history including questions about if, when, and how the patient has fallen. Falling in the past year makes a patient statistically likely to fall in the current year. The patient should be asked how he felt after the fall. The reported loss of consciousness or memory calls for probing for a stroke, seizure, or cardiac arrhythmia as a cause.

The physical examination tests gait, balance, reflexes, and leg strength. Diagnosis for diseases and conditions that can affect motor skills like Parkinson's is important, as is probing for "orthostatic hypotension," a plunge in blood pressure upon standing. Orthostatism can reflect a correctable mix of interacting medications including antidepressants, blood pressure pills, sedatives, antipsychotics, and diuretics. Or, it can reveal "hypovolemia," reduced blood volume caused by dehydration or internal bleeding.

The Mayo Clinic (among others) has identified eleven "Risk Factors for Falls":

1. Lower Extremity Weakness
2. History of Falls
3. Gait Deficit
4. Balance Deficit
5. Use of Assistive Device*
6. Visual Defect
7. Impaired Activities of Daily Living
8. Depression
9. Cognitive Impairment
10. Age ≥ 80 years
11. Multiple medications.

When patients do not present in the clinic or hospital with obvious risk factors, that is not the end of the story; there are other

---

* Such as a cane, wheelchair, or walker.

good clinical indicators of falls. The patient's complaints of a mobility problem statistically predicts a fall, as does the observation that he cannot rise from a chair without gripping the arms, or walks from the waiting room with an uneven gait. But in today's corporate clinics with rigidly rationed interview minutes, the doctor might not have the chance to see the transition from the waiting area to the exam room, or to receive a volunteered complaint. Instead he can ask the patient to perform brief and telling physical exercises. Failure to "tandem stand" with the toe of one foot touching the heel of the other for ten seconds predicts falling, as does the inability to tandem stand and then walk two meters with heel touching toe. The "get up and go" test shows that the patient is likely to fall if he cannot walk ten meters in thirteen seconds. Note that these tests take mere *seconds*. Even the most industrial, profit-centered HMO clinic or office should provide them.

The Centers for Disease Control and Prevention now recommends five preventative measures for older people, all of which should be implemented by their clinical providers to keep them as safe as possible:

1. Regular exercise, which helps with balance, strength, and above all, mobility.
2. Ambulatory patients should have their medications reviewed to determine if they are at risk for drug interactions that could make them unsteady, dizzy, or lose balance.
3. Patients should have annual eye exams, since vision deficits lead to falls.
4. They should have their homes or institutional environments assessed for hazards and improved. Minimal "fall proofing" means replacing dim lighting, especially on stairs, and plugging in night-lights. It involves removing obstacles and tripping hazards, placing grab bars around toilets and in showers, and tacking down carpets. Since 70 percent of falls

happen in homes, minor mindful maintenance or corrective carpentry amounts to medicine.

5. Vitamin D supplements should be taken not simply to help harden bones, but also to increase muscle strength, a newly found benefit.

In 2007, the *Journal of the American Medical Association* published a landmark meta-analysis on the efficacy of fall screening and prevention studies called "Will My Patient Fall?" In addition to describing statistically rated predictive tools, *JAMA* reported that "multifactorial interventions" (such as the five-part CDC bundle) reduced the falling rates of older Americans by 30 to 40 percent.

So what should a patient or his advocate do? The simple answer is to ask to be screened for falling risks, and reveal your fall history and mobility issues. If you are at risk, insist on getting a fall-prevention bundle, as well as fall education which now exists in a variety of electronic and printed forms and teaches a host of safe techniques, as well as salient facts including that more falls occur going downstairs than going upstairs, and 35 percent of hip fractures occur at night, hence use a night-light.

Falls plague hospitals and nursing homes (now optimistically called long-term care facilities). Studies suggest that about half of all nursing home patients fall each year. The fact that many of these people suffer from dementia makes them difficult to educate about prevention. They must be protected, which requires adequate staff to watch them. Usually the result of inattention, if only for short periods, most nursing home falls are medical errors.

Falls in acute care hospitals range from 1.3 to 8.9 per 1,000 patient days. Around the world the average rate is about 3 per 1,000 hospital days. Falls never should happen in hospitals. When they do, they almost always constitute medical errors. Falls vary across specialties and peak in wards housing geriatric, neurological, and rehabilitation patients requiring heightened scrutiny.

Medicare's No Pay for Errors List includes "fall or trauma resulting in serious injury," which blocks government insurance from funding care for about one out of five of these accidents. Fearing this complication and having to eat its costs, many hospitals screen for fall risks on admission.

One widely-adopted measure called STRATIFY (St. Thomas Risk Assessment Tool in Falling for Elderly In-patients) uses a simple five-part questionnaire that predicts with statistical accuracy if a patient is immediately at risk for falling. It asks:

1.   Did the patient present to hospital with a fall or has he or she fallen in the ward since admission?
      (Yes= 1, No=0)

2.   Do you think patient is agitated?
      (Yes= 1, No=0)

3.   Visually impaired to the extent that everyday function is affected?
      (Yes= 1, No=0)

4.   In need of frequent toileting?
      (Yes= 1, No=0)
      Transfer and mobility score of 3 or 4?*
      Total score =

Based on studies reported in the *British Medical Journal* in 1997, the overall STRATIFY score is less important than having two or more "yes" answers, which signifies that the hospitalized

---

* Transfer (from bed to chair) is scored as follows: 0, unable; 1, major help needed; 2, minor help; 3, independent. For mobility: 0, immobile; 1, independent with a wheelchair; 2, walks with help of one person; 3, independent.

patient has a 50–50 chance of falling in the next week. Once identified as a fall risk, the patient rapidly should become the target of careful attention: bedside signs, high visibility "alert" wristbands, specialized footwear, computer-generated education packets at the "consumer" level, and chair *and* bed alarms. Since toileting is so dangerous—it produces upwards of 40 percent of crashes in some hospitals—the function is specifically scheduled and planned down to the number of nurses supervising and the type of equipment (bed pan, bedside commode, etc.). Each at-risk patient is provided with a rigorous medication review to guard against dysfunctional "polypharmacy" (multiple prescriptions with interactions), vision vetting, and assessment for assistive devices (walkers, crutches, etc.). In large multi-hospital studies with thousands of patients, intervention groups with bundled preventative measures had about 30 percent less falls than in-patient control groups getting the usual care according to a 2013 report in the *Annals of Internal Medicine* supported by AHRQ.

Other measures have been found to work in certain hospitals. One key is staff re-training and education. In particular, interdisciplinary fall teams with "clinical champions" identify potential victims and hazards, circulate data on existing and prevented accidents, and above all according to the *Annals*, "change the prevailing nihilistic attitude that falls are 'inevitable' and 'nothing can be done.'"

Further, most patients should be intensively educated on using call buttons and other help-seeking measures available including "alert" wristbands. To the extent possible, binders like restraints and catheters should be avoided. Urinary tract infections lead to frequent toileting, which then leads to falls, and should be addressed aggressively. For those prone to falling out of bed, bed rails sometimes work, but putting the bed on the floor is a far superior fix, especially in long-term care.

Some studies have shown the efficacy of high-tech plastic hip protectors as a measure for defending frail and elderly beset with balance problems. Unfortunately the largest and best-funded research on the tool was seriously flawed. The controversy over hip pads grew out of a huge study performed by the medical schools at Harvard University, Washington University in St. Louis, and the University of Maryland under the auspices of the National Institute of Aging of NIH that drew from 37 nursing homes in Boston, Baltimore, and St. Louis. Over a thousand participants, average age 85, wore a hip protector only on one side. The devices were slim energy-deflecting shells that tucked into sleeves in undergarments. The researchers felt that they had cleverly discerned a way around the flaw in most big studies—namely that patients in control and intervention groups do not have identical experiences, while the musculoskeletal structure of the same individual does. So each patient was his or her own control group. The study concluded after twenty months and the authors announced that the hip pads had no measurable effect; protected hips were as likely to be fractured as unprotected ones.

Unfortunately, the authors of the article which appeared in the *Journal of the American Medical Association* in 2007 "were not forthcoming with providing information" requested by the editors that having only one protector altered gait and made the patients tend to "fall to the protected side."

Consequently the study was investigated by the federal Office for Human Research Protection of the Department of Health and Human Services and found ethically inadequate for failing to warn participants of the risks. Today, online versions of the journal article bear an onerous official caveat that "An Expression of Concern about this Article has been published."

Too clever by half, and arguably unethical, the 37-nursing home study still left the profession with the notions that hip pads are controversial and ineffective. In fact, prudent geriatric professionals do well to prescribe them "bilaterally" to the frail elderly, and especially to women with a history of falls. Pads do no harm, and some evidence reflects that they protect against hip fractures that can be life-ending, life-shortening, and damaging milestones.

Another fall strategy that evidently works (at least in small studies at single institutions) is "post-mortems," which basically means collecting, analyzing, and disclosing evidence about falls. Hospital floors that count and post fall statistics often see the numbers go down from month to month. Some larger well-funded hospitals now utilize multi-disciplinary teams that review all falls, perform "root cause analyses," and publicize the findings. Virginia Mason Hospital in Seattle actually established a unit it calls "Falls University" to accomplish these tasks (with a steady and consistent drop in falls). In addition, it has pharmacists examine every fall to see if there was a link between the patient's medication and the accident.

What can patients and their advocates do to avoid these deadly and disruptive traumas? First, they should ask to be screened for falls. Most institutions should provide a structured point-scoring interview based on STRATIFY or the similar Morse Falls Scale (MFS). If a patient cannot be formally screened, he should tell his care provider his history of falling or concerns about mobility. If he is unsure if he is at risk, he should perform a tandem standing or walking test (in the presence of a spotter). Many otherwise healthy elderly will be surprised to discover how difficult they will find these simple exams and to learn that they are vulnerable. If there is any indication of being at risk, the patient or his advocate should ask for fall protections (hopefully a bundle of them) to be implemented. Falls while in institutional care are brutal, tragic, plentiful, and avoidable medical errors.

CHAPTER THIRTEEN: The Health-Care Environment Should Be Clean and Rational

Although he has yet to appear in standard medical histories, Earle H. Spaulding, who died in 1995 at 88, probably is the most influential modern preventer of introgenic disease. After receiving a doctorate from Yale in 1936 in what was then called bacteriology, Spaulding moved to Temple University Medical School in Philadelphia. During his lifetime and leadership, the field became known as microbiology as it grew to encompass non-bacterial bits like fungi, viruses, and prions (the misfolded protein fragments that cause deadly transmissible spongiform encephalopathies including Mad Cow disease).

While teaching at Temple, Spaulding headed the university hospital's pathology lab, wrote the seminal *Manual of Clinical Microbiology*, authored over a hundred papers on microbes, and battled outbreaks and epidemics in diverse communities and institutions. Spaulding drilled Temple medical and microbiology students on disinfection and sterilization measures. In the early days, the subject lacked the glamor of heroic surgical techniques and curing diseases like polio, but Spaulding persisted. He taught 200 students at a clip, memorized all of their names, hosted weekly brown-bag lunches featuring his wife's famous baked goods, became the school's best loved professor, and developed generations of infection fighters.

While disinfection and sterilization had been practiced for centuries, Spaulding knew that they had not been systematically studied. Worse, cleaning behaviors and compounds often had no or even dysfunctional effects that spread disease or caused disasters. For instance, when sodium hypochlorite, the salt found in common bleach, comes in contact with urine or vomit a toxic gas can be released.

During an intense fifteen-year span that began shortly after his arrival at Temple, Spaulding tested every available germicide and fungicide against dangerous microbes to determine what worked, what did not, and what bruised the environment. In addition to publishing his results, Spaulding in the 1950s and '60s conceptualized an antimicrobial framework. He provided a rational paradigm for patient care surfaces and equipment that a half century later in 2008 the CDC called "so clear and logical that it has been retained, refined, and successfully used by infection control professionals and others when planning methods for disinfection or sterilization."

Disinfection, by the way, means killing most disease-causing pathogens and other micro-organisms by chemical or physical means. It may not eliminate spores—the dried out, hardened "defensive" forms of bacteria like *C. diff.* Sterilization ideally achieves a state free of all living organisms including spores, but often is more theoretical than actual. The CDC defines it as "a probability function" as in "the probability of a micro-organism surviving sterilization being one in a million."

THE SPAULDING PARADIGM

Contact Point	Disinfection Required	Device Class
Sterile body cavity	Sterilization	Critical
Mucous membranes	High level	Semi-critical
Intact skin	Low level	Non-critical

In Spaulding's approach, "critical" items include urinary and cardiac catheters, surgical tools, implants, ultrasound probes, and any other items that invade sterile tissue, body cavities, and the vascular system. Because any microbial contamination could spawn disease, this equipment must be sterilized rigorously to be free even of spores.

A few items such as sutures can be purchased sterile and used once. But most tools that enter and emerge from tissue have to be re-sterilized, often in an autoclave, a pressurized steam cabinet heated to 250° Fahrenheit. Heat-sensitive items like endoscopes (flexible tubes with optical systems) must be treated with chemical sterilants approved by the Food and Drug Administration. Spaulding and his successors tested these compounds to establish specific contact time, concentration, and pH (degree of acidity or alkalinity). While kind to equipment, low-temperature sterilization causes a range of risks from explosions to eye and skin damage, convulsions, and spontaneous abortions, so the process must be handled with extreme care.

A major breakthrough occurred in 1993 with the marketing of sterilization chambers using non-toxic hydrogen peroxide gas plasma. Regarded as the fourth state of matter (after solids, liquids, and gases) plasmas activated by radio or microwaves contain "free radicals," atoms with unpaired electrons that invade cells, disrupt their nuclear DNA, and slaughter them.

Whether chemical or physical, sterilization carries risks. But Spaulding found that not all tools need complete microbial annihilation, including those that touch non-intact skin and mucous membranes, which are rows of joined epithelial (surface) cells that secrete sticky fluids in body cavities that come in contact with the air in the eyes, nose, mouth, throat, lungs, gut, and genitals. Known as "semi-critical" items, these include anesthesia and respiratory tubes, cystoscopes, laryngoscopes, and rectal catheters among others. They call for a meticulous cleaning followed by disinfection with approved FDA liquids that may leave spores behind. Such compounds include glutaraldehyde, which is used as a common cleanser of dental equipment, in wart removal, and as a biocide in hydraulic fracturing (fracking), and peracetic acid (commonly used as a bathroom cleaner and beverage pasteurizer).

In health care, "noncritical" items come in contact with intact skin, generally a staunch barrier against infection. This equipment comes in two types: patient care tools like crutches, walkers, bed pans, and blood pressure cuffs; and environmental surfaces such as tables, drapes, walls, floors, windows, and appliances. Most non-critical items can be cleaned where used and do not require central decontamination.

Non-critical items pose the threat of "secondary transmission" of infection via the hands of health care workers or medical equipment that touches multiple patients. The CDC guidelines include low-level disinfectants like ethyl or isopropyl alcohol, sodium hypochlorite (bleach) phenolic (coal tar) compounds, iodophers (iodine plus detergents), and ammonium germicides all in recommended concentrations and with contact times of twenty to sixty seconds in contrast to high-level disinfection which takes about twelve minutes. The province of housekeeping or "environmental services," such cleaning can do away with bacteria like salmonella, *E. coli*, fungi, and yeasts.

A mundane albeit critical pursuit, housekeeping has not been studied much from a scientific standpoint. Those who perform it may be on staff at a hospital, or the service can be outsourced. Some infectious disease experts favor hired cleaning staff over contractors, since the latter adhere to rigid work terms and may be less responsive during off-peak hours or, worse, during outbreaks. In-house domestic cleaners probably can be trained more thoroughly on neglected and difficult pieces like drip stands and electrical equipment.

Some duties, especially spot-cleaning of certain surfaces in patient rooms, fall to nursing. Other often touched items like trays and utensils "belong" to the dietary staff. Crutches, canes, and walkers are the bailiwick of physical therapy, which can clean them or not. Gurneys and transports show up from a variety of departments like surgery or radiology. So it is difficult to track who cleans what, and frankly some surfaces simply fall between the cracks. Items that do not get cleaned can become "reservoirs" of MRSA, *C. diff.* and other pathogens that spawn hospital-acquired infections.

Cleaning methods and compounds also have ups and downs. Detergent-based wipes and mopping may remove microbes, but also spread them to other surfaces and rooms. Rules of thumb hold that a wipe wipes a single piece of equipment, that mop water should be changed after fifteen minutes, and that mop heads must be laundered daily. Disinfectants, especially common chlorine-based ones, do an effective job on most pathogens but they pit surfaces and equipment leaving niches for new bacteria, and they cause environmental harm when they flow out of the hospital.

The CDC has well worked out, studied, and proven guidelines for safely cleaning, disinfecting, and/or sterilizing endoscopes, bronchoscopes, biopsy forceps, laparoscopes, tonometers (human pressure gauges), cervical diaphragm fitting rings, dental instruments, hemodialysis equipment, endocavity probes, cryosurgical instruments, colonoscopy devices, thermometers, and numerous other instruments and environments. The Agency publishes protocols for items contaminated with Hepatitis B virus, Hepatitis C, HIV, tuberculosis, human papillomavirus (HPV), *C. diff*, *E. coli*, and cryptosporidium (a protozoa that causes diarrhea), norovirus (a non-enveloped RNA strand that causes high fever and cramps), severe acute respiratory syndrome (SARS), *Heliobacter pylori (a cause* of gastric ulcers), rotovirus (a double-stranded RNA that gives infants and young children grueling diarrhea), Ebola, and even possible bio-terrorist agents such as anthrax, plague, smallpox, and arena virus. The CDC also guides health-care facilities on decontaminating spills of blood and bodily substances, plants, pests, floors, carpets, laundry, bedding, and on controlling the transmission of air and waterborne diseases.

Comprehensive air standards address heating, cooling, ventilation, exhausts, false ceilings, windows, building materials, elevators, vacuums, and heliports. Unless these guidelines are followed, a host of diseases can spread including tuberculosis, streptococcus, staphylococcus, influenza, measles and adenoviruses (a source of respiratory distress, conjunctivitis, and multiple organ failure), and aspergillus, a fungus that causes sinusitis as well as abscesses in the brain, kidneys, lungs, liver, and spleen.

Water, the lifeblood of health-care facilities, plays a role in surgery, sanitation, labs, and hygiene. CDC guidelines apply to equipment like cooling towers, condensers, boilers, pipe connections with municipal systems, ice-makers, and hydrotherapy tanks. The CDC has measures to prevent reservoirs of pathogens like *Legionella*, pseudomonas, and acinetobacter (a source of urinary and bloodstream infections and iatrogenic pneumonia) from forming in hospital potable water, dialysis water, holy water, endoscope reprocessors, bathtubs, faucet aerators, sinks, showers, dental unit water lines, eyewash stations, and toilets. Some of these measures seem fairly simple. For instance, endoscope reprocessing chemicals should be rinsed with alcohol then dried with forced air. Bathtubs should be drained and disinfected after every use. Faucet aerators, a significant source of *Legionella*, require monthly cleaning and disinfection, and if *Legionella* is sampled they can be thrown away. Significant sources of pseudomonas, sinks should be segregated into ones for hand washing, and others for flushing contaminated fluids.

During the celebration of the U.S. Bicentennial in 1976, an unknown pneumonia and flu-like condition struck 221 American Legion military veterans in a Philadelphia hotel, killing thirty-four. The lethal waterborne bacteria had colonized in the hotel air-conditioning system. The scourge became known as Legionnaire's Disease and the germ as *Legionella*.

Naturally occurring, *Legionella* is not generally a mortal threat to healthy young people with intact immune systems. However, it can wreak havoc on institutionalized elderly and immunocompromised patients. Most Americans probably have heard about outbreaks in local hospitals or nursing homes. These public-health crises kill upwards of 20 percent of infected victims. Outbreaks of *Legionella*, and other waterborne bacterial diseases, are serious medical errors that largely can be prevented. According to the CDC, cold water stored below 68°F (20°C) is hostile to these germs. Hot water should be kept above 140°F (60°C) and returned to tanks at or above 124°F (51°C). Since 140° is scaldingly hot, institutional plumbing should place mixing valves near shower-heads and faucets. Hospital water and patient fluids can be cultured routinely for *Legionella*. When found, the system can be flushed with chlorine compounds, ionic forms of silver and copper, or super-heated to near boiling. Likewise, major structures like boilers, cooling towers, and condensers, should be scrubbed then "shocked" with high heat and/or hyperchlorination to prevent outbreaks.

Most Americans probably would be surprised to learn that CDC standards for disinfection and sterilization in health-care facilities lack legal force. Obviously, these standards should be enforceable as laws or regulations by federal or state agencies. In fact they are, but in only two small after-the-fact ways. If there is an outbreak of a disease like *Legionella*, tuberculosis, or Hepatitis B or C, the CDC (or state health department) may gather evidence and/or direct the clean-up and remediation. Also, many of the sterilants, disinfectants, and detergents recommended by CDC are registered with the Environmental Protection Agency under a statute called the Federal Insecticide, Fungicide, and Rodenticide Act (FIFRA) that mandates label directions on chemical compatibility, safe uses, shelving, and disposal. Under FIFRA, a user who flouts the label directions causing injury assumes liability and may be fined or even imprisoned.

One can be under no illusion that Washington in its weak anti-regulatory mood will enact the rest of the extensive guidelines into law, even though they provide a detailed framework for clean, rational infection-free conditions that are totally in the interest of everyone cared for or working in hospitals, clinics, and nursing homes. So what should patients and their advocates do? At a minimum, before or upon admission to an acute or long-term care facility they should ask whether CDC guidelines will be followed, since these standards are well-known, evidence-based, and tantamount to best practices. The answer in a hospital that vows adherence to patient-centered care may be "yes," but such a response also may be expedient, superficial, and calculated simply to put the patient in a bed and start billing him.

Here is what I suggest. When you sign your financial responsibility form authorizing payment through insurance or otherwise, or when you provide your informed consent to procedures, medication, and supplying data you should write: "all CDC guidelines on infection, prevention, and control will be followed." Ask the person presenting you with the hospital's form to sign this simple added language. If he asks which guidelines, show him the current official list on the CDC's website: http://www.cdc.gov/HAI/prevent/prevent_pubs.html. Note that the trademark of the Centers for Disease Control is "CDC 24/7: Saving Lives. Protecting People."

You are highly vulnerable in a hospital or nursing facility. The essential reason why these places are more dangerous than your residence is that there are no outbreaks of disease in homes. In the hospital, your life may be at stake and you need protection. One way to get it is by making the CDC standards as contractual between the provider and patient as are the payment stream and the written informed consent to treatment.

Basically dirt removal, housekeeping unfortunately remains the lowest job in the hospital. Yet, in the end, frank fear of infection, of bugs, and superbugs, of failing antibiotics that promote rather than quell outbreaks, and of cross-contamination from patient to patient sometimes with the hands, gloves, gowns, gauges and tools of health-care workers as vectors, should cause patients and their families to demand not to be in a dirty (i.e., dangerous) hospital, clinic, or nursing home. By the same token, there probably is no reason to worry over a stained carpet on a family lounge floor (although it might be more sanitary to have moppable tiles) or some momentary street dirt from shoes under a patient's bed. Such flaws generally have not been found to lead to outbreaks of disease.

Moreover, in a hospital, all that glitters is not gold. Microbes associated with MRSA, *C. diff.* and Vancomycin-resistant enterococci are invisible and can linger in the environment for weeks. The same can be said for flu, norovirus, and fungi like *Candida albicans* that infect the gut, genitals, and skin. Coliform (intestinal) bacteria such as *E. coli* and klebisella can survive on wet or dry surfaces for long periods. The general rule is that pathogens persist unless removed by cleansing. They get onto hands, rise with dust, or attach to moisture droplets before settling on ledges, linen, shelves, curtains, telephones, and medical equipment.

Some common germs like pseudomonas spread in wet areas such as sinks and showers. *C. diff.* and VRE contaminate commodes. MRSA floats onto rarely cleaned surfaces like keyboards. Klebisella and other coliforms contaminate mops, buckets, and bowls. Beds and surfaces near them offer the highest hazards to patients. Risk rises dramatically when patients are admitted to rooms where the prior occupant was infected or colonized with pathogens. Wide flat surfaces often get cleaned, but small finicky ones like buttons and switches receive little attention, a fate also reserved for patient clothes lockers, the tops of cabinets, and perhaps most notoriously the underside of the over-bed tables. Post-cleaning inspection with illuminometers (handheld consoles that can detect the bioluminescence of left behind organic materials like bacteria and mold) can help determine if more work needs to be done, but these units that have proven successful in the food industry seem underutilized, perhaps because they light up a lot of safe biologicals; plus the price can approach three thousand dollars. Even so, bioluminescent inspections and the threat of them has been shown to stimulate staff to more thoroughness.

Special care units require special care and common sense. Disinfectants should not be used on or in incubators or bassinettes while babies occupy them. After an infant leaves, these can be decontaminated with a phenolic (coal tar) disinfectant, rinsed with tap water and dried before the next baby arrives. In a cardiac intensive care unit, a notorious outbreak occurred when blood pressure monitors were coated with mists from nearby cleaning water, leading to open heart surgery patients becoming septic. In general, ICUs and other units involving debilitated and immune-suppressed patients need greater rigor and scrutiny from housekeeping.

For all the heightened attention to cleaning, disinfection, and sterilization in acute care, there is an equal measure of disappointment that has started to dampen enthusiasm for the Spaulding scheme. In a 2011 study the CDC reported that 722,000 hospitalized Americans contracted hospital infections, and 75,000 died. A widely reported study of thirty-six acute care hospitals showed that less than half of high-risk surfaces tagged with fluorescent markers had been cleaned at discharge and before a new patient took occupancy. These rooms had failed what has become known as "terminal disinfection" or TDI.

The Spaulding scheme focused on "trees"—the critical and semi-critical items that penetrated bodies—not the "forests" of health care, the rooms and surfaces that comprise hospitals.

Unfortunately those surfaces and the people who touch them—health-care professionals, cleaners, and technicians—become conduits for multiple drug-resistant organisms (MDROS) that when spread and ingested even in minute quantities make already sick people much sicker. Studies also proved that assignment to a room of a prior patient colonized or infected with MDROS, whether MRSA, VRE, *C. diff*, pseudomonas, or acenetobacteria, gave the new occupant a greatly heightened risk of catching the germ. For added measure, the CDC reported that its guidelines for "reprocessing" (e.g. the technical disinfection and sterilization of critical and semi-critical pieces such as endoscopes) were not being followed "and outbreaks of infection continue to occur." Recall that the CDC lacks enforcement powers to rectify lax practices.

Obviously, patients cannot observe the workings of autoclaves and gas plasma chambers. Nor can they know whether the probe that will enter their body has had adequate contact time with a chemical sterilant. But they do see and fear their rooms, and that has bred powerful movements in favor of terminal disinfection (TDI) and no-touch disinfection (NDI).

Terminal disinfection basically involves intensive cleaning and evaluation of all "high touch" surfaces—not walls or windows—every time a patient is discharged from a room. The CDC reports that disease transmission is reduced substantially when comprehensive room disinfection is coupled with monitoring for remaining pathogens by taking swab or agar slide cultures (both slow to produce results) or with fluorescent gels or bioluminescence (which are immediate). Visual or "direct examination," the usual cheap method employed by the housekeeping or environmental service crews, has no value since the naked eye cannot perceive microbes.

Checklists have become indispensable to surgical safety, central line catheters, and respirator practice, but none is more important than the one reporting terminal disinfection of the patient's room. What follows is the CDC's checklist. Every hospital should have something similar and provide it upon request to the patient or his advocate. If possible, the patient should refuse a room if he cannot be given the checklist. Obviously, a consumer can obtain something like this when buying a car. One's safety is at least equally at stake in a hospital.

CDC Environmental Checklist for Monitoring Terminal Cleaning

Date:		
Unit:		
Room Number:		
Initials of ES staff (optional):		

Evaluate the following: priority sites for each patient room:

High-touch Room Surfaces	Cleaned	Not Cleaned	Not Present in Room
Bed tails / controls			
Tray table			
N pole (21" ab area)			
Call box / button			
Telephone			
Bedside table handle			
Chair			
Room sink			
Room light switch			

Room inner door knob			
Bathroom inner door knob / plate			
Bathroom light switch			
Bathroom handrails by toilet			
Bathroom sink			
Toilet seat			
Toilet flush handle			
Toilet bedpan cleaner			

Evaluate the following additional sites if these equipment are present in the room:

High-touch Room Surfaces	Cleaned	Not Cleaned	Not Present in Room
IV pump control			
Multi-module monitor controls			
Multi-module monitor touch screen			
Multi-module monitor cables			
Ventilator control panel			

Mark the monitoring method used:

____Direct observation   ____Fluorescent gel

____Swab cultures   ____ATP system

____Agar slide cultures

Upon receiving a checklist, a patient or advocate should consider refusing the room if all high touch surfaces have not been cleaned, or if the only monitoring method is limited to direct observation (i.e., visual inspection). They also should ask for the immediate infectious history of the room. In other words, was the person who previously used the bed and bathroom suffering from *C. diff,* MRSA, VRE, or some other multiple drug-resistant organism? If so, the chances of contracting such germs are sufficiently elevated that it would make sense to wait for another room. This is a process that is not always possible given a patient's dire condition requiring immediate treatment or the lack of available beds. However, it might be reasonable to take the bed if a previous patient who had a hospital-acquired infection provided that the room has been put through no-touch disinfection as an adjunct to, but not a substitute for, serious terminal cleaning.

Today one of the good ways that hospitals have begun to market and compete on a technology basis is whether they offer NDI, which comes in a variety of forms. The major types include foggers and sprayers that dispense hydrogen peroxide as an aerosol or vapor, and robots emitting ultraviolet radiation. Both have been successful in laboratory settings and emerging data also suggest clinical efficacy. Hydrogen peroxide systems have been effective at removing pathogen reservoirs, including at Johns Hopkins where the spray coats every surface, oxidizes the germs and spores, and then breaks down harmlessly into water and oxygen. The rooms and vents must be rigorously sealed during the treatment, which is popular with staff who are encouraged to bring all their computers, stethoscopes and other gear inside for safe decontamination. At Hopkins a vapor sprayer reduced MDRO infection by 64 percent.

UV radiation also reduces pathogens (by degrading their DNA) although not as completely as spraying, since the germs must be in the robot's line of sight. In a major study published in the *American Journal of Infection Control*, a pulsed xenon ultra-violet machine reduced MDRO and *C. diff.* rates by 20 percent during a twenty-two-month period when UV radiation was used over eleven thousand times at Westchester Hospital in Valhalla, New York. At almost $80,000, a UV robot costs about twice as much as the H_2O_2 technology, yet UV now is used far more frequently. In fact, over 250 hospitals, including the Department of Veteran Affairs, use it. Why? UV is somewhat simpler to operate and rooms may be closed off but not meticulously sealed. However, the real reason is cycle time. It takes two to three hours to gas a hospital room with H_2O_2 but only minutes to zap it with UV, perhaps somewhat longer if the robot is placed at multiple points to shoot rays.

These machines have science fiction appeal. The H_2O_2 sprayer looks like the chubby dancing Droid from TV commercials, while the UV robot resembles R2-D2 from *Star Wars*. Both seem enormously promising and will go through additional studies and refinement, and both have similar drawbacks. Sub-lethal dosing with H_2O_2 could cause already tough pathogens to develop increased tolerance. Likewise, ultraviolet is known to be mutagenic, and the radiation—especially if emitted from weakening bulbs—could produce resistant strains.

In my region, the dominant hospital system has acquired two new pulsed xenon ultraviolet machines whose necks extend eerily upward before the contraptions, both nicknamed "Violet," click and shoot beams twenty-five times brighter than sunlight. Patients reportedly are delighted to see Violet since they want to be safe, and hope to get well rather than sicker from rooms with pathogens that the robot zaps away.

In the future, patient rooms, operating rooms, ICU's and emergency departments may become self-sterilizing (although not self-cleaning) with permanent foggers, sprayers, germ zappers and hermetic sealing systems. In fact, to some extent this process already is occurring by coating or impregnating surfaces with silver or copper, germicides, or antimicrobial substances activated by light.

The anti-disease qualities of heavy metals like lead, mercury, gold, and silver have been known since ancient times. Silver-coated medical instruments have utility today, and silver particles are sometimes mixed with H_2O_2 vapor. Ionized copper in patient care surfaces leads to microbial cell death by damaging lipids, DNA, and proteins. Copper and silver electrostatically limit *Legionella* in hospital water systems and aspergillus in building materials. Important recent research showed that copper-laced surfaces in an ICU reduced infection by more than 50 percent.

Other heavy metals including titanium are being studied for surface infection control, as are germicides such as the pervasive and controversial compound triclosan, found in toothpastes and antimicrobial soaps, and cellulose acetate layering including photosensitizers. Surfacing is significant and delicate work especially because of interactions with other systems. For instance the chlorine, ammonium, and alcohol-based fluids approved by the EPA can degrade some of these materials, scarring surfaces and leaving nooks and crannies for pathogen reservoirs to form. As for triclosan, when hit by UV rays it emits poisonous dioxins.

■

Besides developing infection controls, health-care facilities can become sensible hence safer in other ways. Hospitals and nursing homes in some respects had to become more rational in the twentieth century due to declining availability of land. Older institutions sprawled out of homes or charitable buildings on vast tracts. Usually low-rise, they sometimes came to cover many blocks with poor interconnections and long, confusing transits for patients and families involving multiple sets of stairs and elevator banks, tunnels, and bridges to different buildings. Before World War II, less land availability led to vertical construction patterns. High-rise hospitals had more compact floors, and most internal voyaging was done on elevators.

In many places, long and dangerous wheelchair and gurney rides for sedated or intravenously hooked-up patients remain problems that can be aggravated if transit is assigned to low-level aides untrained in what to do if the patient has a setback. Rational hospitals plan for such emergencies either by recognizing that these shuttles are important tasks worthy of skilled nurses or by ensuring ready communications and immediate access to medical care wherever the transport might be. Simply parking a patient unattended while he awaits an x-ray or test should be prohibited.

Maze-like, chaotically organized acute and long-term care institutions with many wings, floors, exits, office areas, parking lots, and labs remain problematic for ambulatory patients, particularly demented ones who tend to get lost, hurt in falls, and exposed to the elements. Staff simply cannot watch them at all times. One popular fix is to microchip plastic patient bracelets to GPS systems, allowing wanderers to be located instantly. What is good enough for pets surely should be good enough for patients.

The modern hospital environment also can be constructed or reconstructed more conducively to reduce medical errors, increase safety, and improve outcomes. For a long time, a gamut of features necessary to upgrade acute care became known in the health care and building trades as "The Fable Hospital" or, as renovations began being completed, as "The Fable Hospital 2.0."

After the millennium, an influential private reform group, the Institute for Healthcare Improvement of Cambridge, Massachusetts announced a campaign to save 100,000 lives with "evidence based design" as one of its cornerstones, and over 4,000 hospitals subscribed to the idea. The renovations of the period saw hospitals grow hotel-like with construction costs approaching $500 per square foot, and amenities including lavish lobbies, gyms, plantscaping, art, cafes, and other features collectively known as "hospitality elements."

But the changes also required "environmental interventions" supported by research. Above all, these pointed to single patient rooms. Studies showed that these units reduced hospital-acquired infections, improved patient sleep, satisfaction, privacy, and family and staff communications while reducing medical errors, falls, and stress. Single rooms even raised staff effectiveness and satisfaction, which might seem paradoxical given the presumed ease of treating two patients in one space. Regardless, the research is clear that a patient or advocate should ask for a single room, and perhaps other factors being equal choose an acute or long-term facility based on the availability of private lodging.

Other research findings included putting a "family zone" with bedding in an alcove in the single room. Not only did that elevate mood, but it also reduced falls. Additional reforms included making rooms "acuity adaptable" or, in other words, able to upgrade to intensive care without moving the patient. Doing so reduced falls, and errors, and increased satisfaction for staff while lessening their injuries. Similarly, there was especially strong evidence that using ceiling-hung alifts in patients' rooms and baths reduced staff injuries. Touches like carpeting, noise-reducing finishes, natural views, and improved lighting, which reduced errors, falls, pain, depression, and even length of stay, were far more than atmospheric as research documented in the *Journal of Healthcare Management* in 2013 shows.

∎

Another major progressive theme includes human-factors engineering (or ergonomics), which has been adapted from the automotive industry to keep people from hurting themselves. For instance, a transmission can't be put in reverse unless the driver's foot is on the brake. These automatic checks that prevent mistakes are known as "forcing functions" and slowly they are being shifted to health care. Anesthesia and pain control are somewhat in the lead. For example, patient-controlled analgesis pumps have been engineered to block overdoses. Prescribed anesthesia canisters cannot receive tubes except from the person awaiting surgery. Too often other tubes look alike and can be inserted in the wrong patient port. For instance, a chest tube and feeding tube are quite similar and crossing them can prove fatal.

During 2010 congressional hearings on medical errors, Senator Kay Hagan (D-NC) became incredulous while listening to Peter Pronovost's frightening testimony that different types of catheters lacked unique connection points and could be mixed up. She asked "how it was possible we had figured how to make diesel fuel nozzles that don't fit gas-powered cars, but we can't figure out how to make different catheter connections so doctors don't place patients in harm's way."

To Pronovost it was a "perfect analogy" for the unsafe medical environment. Hagen, of course, was right. A patient should be as safe as an automobile's gas tank. While the acute care environment is getting better and less hazardous in some ways, it remains risky and thoughtless in others. Some changes, even obvious ones, are a long way off. In the interim, patients and their advocates must remain vigilant. In particular, they should ask staff to trace every tube before and after insertion back to its point of origin to ensure that the right nutrients and medicine course to the right place.

CHAPTER FOURTEEN: The Health-Care Environment Should Be Open and Overseen

Publicly, health professionals support openness, disclosure, and transparency as the means to expose errors, deal with them, learn from them, train on them, and reduce them. Attend a conference on infections or other medical mistakes, and be assured that the doctor on the dais will swear that "sunshine" is the best disinfectant. While this is true, as was shown in magnificent late twentieth century and millennial studies that unveiled harm and saved lives, the public disclosure of errors has had a brief and spotty history.

In 1863, Florence Nightingale, the English reformer whose innovations revolutionized military nursing during the Crimean War, released a controversial comparative study of death rates in London hospitals. In the early twentieth century, Ernest Amory Codman, a gifted cancer and orthopedic surgeon at the Massachusetts General Hospital (MGH) for whom Codman bone tumors are named, instituted a system for following medical mistakes in treatment and publicizing them to prove his thesis that one out of three hospital patients endures an error. For his efforts, MGH severed Codman's staff privileges in 1914. He later moved to Philadelphia where he helped found the American College of Surgeons' hospital inspection and standardization efforts. Recently MGH opened the Codman Center for Clinical Effectiveness in Surgery in honor of its outcast of a century before.

Until the late twentieth century, little publicizing of poor procedural results or medical errors occurred although some hospitals and health departments kept registries of various types of surgeries and their success rates. While these results might be made known to practitioners they seldom became public. In many cases the information was poorly managed and of marginal use.

A leading registry was kept by the New York Department of Health for heart procedures, particularly coronary artery bypass grafts (CABG). Performed on an urgent or emergency basis in only thirty hospitals, this surgery, called "cabbage" in the trade, creates a shunt (usually from a vein removed from the patient) to bypass a blockage so blood can flow from the aorta to the coronary artery.

Perusing data in the 1980s, David Axelrod, M.D., New York's Commissioner of Health became alarmed because CABG mortality rates among hospitals varied from 1 to 18 percent. Astonishingly, some patients had a one-in-a-hundred chance of dying while others faced odds of almost one in five depending upon which hospital they chose and the surgeon who performed the bypass.

In 1990, the *Journal of the American Medical Association* published the first comparative study of hospitals doing CABG in New York. As with many studies, institutions were able to remain anonymous. However, the same day that the *JAMA* piece was published, Axelrod and the Department of Health boldly released the names of the hospitals to the *New York Times*, resulting in a public furor. How could the venue of surgery so markedly skew the odds of survival?

The media and the public now clamored for "surgeon-specific" data, in other words the names and mortality rates of CABG doctors. This was a bridge too far for the Health Department, which claimed that since individual surgeons performed fewer operations than hospitals, the statistical power would be weaker and their rates would be "misleading." Also the Health Department's Cardiac Advisory Committee (CAC), a body including some of the most eminent heart surgeons in the United States, wanted to protect practitioners' reputations with anonymity. But the statistical power was more than adequate to provide consumers with a meaningful medical choice, as the Long Island paper *Newsday* showed in a suit against the august state agency that forced release of the surgeon-specific data and named names in 1992.

Public disclosures led to profound changes for hospitals, physicians, and patients. For St. Peter's Hospital in Albany the death rate for CABG performed on an emergency basis reached a staggering 26 percent—almost four times the state average for these risky cases. By conducting a searching analysis, the hospital got to the root of the problem: it was not stabilizing patients (in term of blood pressure, respiratory insufficiency, renal failure, and other factors) before bypass. Shamed, it began medically managing cases preoperatively leading to zero deaths in 54 CABG cases in 1993.

Buffalo's Erie County Hospital topped the state with an 18 percent overall bypass death rate in 1989, which led to a probing site visit by the CAC and suspension of CABG surgery in 1990. Erie implemented quality controls and specialized hiring of cardiac-dedicated anesthesiologists, internists, nurses, and bypass technicians under a new permanent full-time chief. Mortality rates plunged in every three-year reporting cycle. By 1993–95 it hit 2.51 percent, which was below the state average of 2.57 percent. In the 1996–1999 time frame, as case numbers climbed from 100 to 219, scrutiny reduced deaths to 1.77 percent.

Winthrop Hospital in Mineola, Long Island took similar steps to drop its 9.2 percent kill rate. After a period on probation, the cardiac surgery program became cohesive, located all functions on one floor, hired a full-time chief, as well as heart-specialized nurses and physician's assistants who teamed to review patients pre-operatively. In 1991, mortality fell to 2.3 percent.

With higher than average overall numbers, Strong Memorial Hospital in Rochester discovered that two surgeons untrained in CABG were operating and raising the death rate. When Strong banned the untrained doctors its rates reduced to normal.

Reporting improved good hospitals as well as bad. Overall, New York CABG deaths fell from 3.52 percent in 1989 to 2.78 percent in 1992. From a public-health perspective, the "risk adjusted mortality rate" (RAMR), which weighs the severity of the patient's illness and other factors like shock, hypertension, and acute myocardial infarction (heart attack) is even more compelling. RAMR dropped 41 percent from 4.17 percent in 1992 to 2.45 percent in 1995 which, according to the Medicare data, topped the nation. By 1999, New York's CABG deaths plunged to the point that patients elsewhere were over 50 percent more likely to die. Other states and hospitals took note, but only California, Massachusetts, New Jersey, Pennsylvania, and the massive Veteran's Health System adopted New York's detailed transparent reporting system, and all saw similar declines in death among CABG patients.

Most controversially, the New York Cardiac Surgery Reporting System disseminated data—known as "report cards"—showing which surgeons were safest and deadliest and in the process proved the correlation between experience and survival. The study looked at all CABG surgeons by volume and divided them into quartiles. Group I operated up to 50 times annually. Group II performed 51 to 100 CABGs; Group III did 101 to 150, and Group IV completed over 150. In 1989 the risk-adjusted mortality rates were 7.94 percent in Group I, 4.5 percent in Group II, 4.05 percent in Group III, and 3.57 percent in Group IV.

With public scrutiny came painful professional assessments, retraining, and departmental reorganizations resulting in all quartiles of surgeons improving by 1991: 3.2 percent in Group I, 2.5 percent in Group II, 2.36 percent in Group III, and 2.45 percent in Group IV. While some critics assumed that a market shift of patients from low-volume to high-volume doctors would occur and account for improvement among the least experienced group, that was not the case, although there was a slight but perceptible movement of medically complex cases from low- to high-volume practitioners.

The prime reason that the low-volume group became statistically safer was that its deadliest seventh—with a risk-adjusted mortality rate of over 16 percent—stopped performing CABG in New York. Some retired, some shifted to other specialties like vascular or general surgery, and others left the state. It is unclear whether any dangerous low-volume surgeons who left New York later performed CABG elsewhere.

Surprisingly, mandatory reporting created only slight changes in market share away from high mortality providers and toward safer hospitals. Perhaps the data remained too complex for the consuming public to fully grasp. Regardless, the real beauties of disclosure were gains in performance, reductions in errors, and drops in mortality. Though the health-care profession and hospitals have not been hurt economically by report cards, they continue to resist them. An especially telling blow came in 2011 when the Society of Thoracic Surgeons—whose superb twenty-five-year Adult Cardiac Surgery Data Base includes patients from 95 percent of heart operating programs in the United States—decided to endorse voluntary rather than mandatory public reporting. So, physicians coping with the greatest killer in the country, heart disease, will publish data as they please that bears upon the population's third greatest killer, medical error.

Published in May of 2014, the 2013 National Healthcare Quality Report by the Agency for Healthcare Research and Quality (AHRQ) constitutes the principal profile of the state of medical care in the United States. The lengthy volume recounts research reflecting that the "rate of harm" associated with hospital stays is 25.1 percent, that the number of "preventable" annual adverse events apart from obstetrical mishaps is 3,023,000, that the thirty-day readmission or "bounceback" rate (a prima facie sign of error) is 14.4 percent, that the yearly bill for "adverse events" excluding obstetrics is $22 billion, and that hospital-error per capita costs average $15,000.

AHRQ finds its mandate, which includes reducing medical error, "complicated by difficulties in ensuring the systematic reporting of patient safety incidents in ongoing protected, consistent, and informative ways. For example, health-care providers fear that if they participate in analysis of patient safety incidents, the findings may be used against them in court or harm their professional reputations." Although data "defined differently across facilities or state lines is fraught with scientific difficulties," AHRC properly lauds as progress that "twenty-seven states have developed voluntary or mandatory reporting systems for, at minimum, serious reportable events . . . that should never happen to a patient."

The statutes vary in quality and in enforcement teeth. Regardless, most providers seem to be evading them, although not necessarily intentionally according to a landmark 2012 national study by U.S. Department of Health and Human Services Inspector General Daniel Levinson entitled "Hospital Reporting Systems Do Not Capture Most Patient Harm." "Most" is an understatement. Levinson's comprehensive study of 189 acute institutions from every state revealed that hospital staffs failed to report fully 86 percent of adverse events. The Inspector General offered two main explanations for the laxity: First, "staff misperceptions about what constitutes patient harm" hardly seems like a credible response from providers who should be able to perceive iatrogenic triggers like infections, medication errors, falls, and bedsores. To their credit, nurses came forward with almost three-quarters of the paltry 14 percent of adverse events that ultimately did get reported.

Second, the Inspector General found that "hospital accreditors reported that in evaluating hospital safety practices, they focus on how event information is used rather than on how it is collected." This is a valuable insight, because hospitals will try to satisfy the agencies whose certificates of approval open the doors to federal and state funds. Since accreditors seem relatively unconcerned with overall reporting compared with highlighting a few serious events as teachable moments, hospitals will follow suit.

Also, the Inspector General is suggesting widespread illegal conduct or at least flouting of federal law, because in order to become a Medicare participant hospitals must hew to "conditions of performance" (COPs in the trade). A key COP requires each hospital to run a Quality Assessment and Performance Improvement (QAPI) program. The QAPI in turn must "track medical errors and adverse patient events, analyze their causes and implement preventive actions and mechanisms that include feedback and learning throughout the hospital."

If you have followed these bureaucratic twists and turns so far, they lead back to what Inspector Levinson was saying about accreditors, whom he also called "surveyors" and "deemers" (Medicare's preferred term). Who are the accreditors? Initially it should be emphasized that we do not have a medical regulation system in this country, we have a certification framework with four main private organizations at the helm.

The most important is the Joint Commission, until recently known as the Joint Commission on Accreditation of Healthcare Organizations (JCAHO) pronounced "Jake O." Nurses and doctors famously used to get their charts in order when Jake O. was coming.

In 1918, the American College of Surgeons (ACS) with Ernest Codman prominent, began the first systematic inspections of hospitals. In 1951, the ACS, the American College of Physicians (ACP), American Hospital Association (AHA), and the American and Canadian Medical Associations created JCAHO, which gained contracts with hospitals and was paid by them to evaluate and certify these institutions.

JCAHO accreditations occurred during three-year cycles. It used to be that visits were scheduled in advance, but unannounced show-ups started about a decade ago. During visits Joint Commission inspectors apply "tracer" methods, meaning that they gather patient charts and follow treatment from admission though discharge. When they spot a gap or error, they summon the nurses and doctors involved, ask questions, and hopefully are satisfied at that moment or over time. Most hospitals win accreditation. In fact, the hospital pass rate is 99 percent.

Accreditation is monetarily meaningful. At its inception in 1965, Medicare's governing organization—then called the Health Care Finance Administration (HCFA)—gave JCAHO its exclusive franchise for deeming. In essence, if JCAHO deemed a hospital accredited, HCFA regarded it as sufficient to receive Medicare and Medicaid funding and presumed it to be compliant with all COPS.

In 2008, after significant errors and safety lapses emerged at accredited hospitals, the federal agency which has changed its name from HCFA to the Centers for Medicare and Medicaid Services (CMS) pulled the Joint Commission's exclusive inspection franchise, and two other private organizations have entered the lucrative field. DNV Healthcare, a unit of the Norwegian risk management conglomerate Det Norske Verite that inspects hospitals worldwide, penetrated the U.S. market. Also, CMS empowered the American Osteopathic Association to inspect hospitals.

The Joint Commission still performs 90 percent of Medicare and Medicaid deeming and even a higher percentage of state accreditations. Under its leader, Mark Chassin, M.D., a nationally recognized quality expert, it has become more safety conscious. Chassin succeeded David Axelrod as Director of the New York Department of Health during the 1990s and guided the Cardiac Reporting Service as it expanded into other procedures beyond by-pass (such as angioplasties) and made it the most transparent system in health-care history. Under Chassin, the Joint Commission has issued and attempted to implement fifteen National

Patient Safety Goals. The goals, which are research-based and make financial sense for constituent hospitals, are as follows:

JOINT COMMISSION NATIONAL PATIENT SAFETY GOALS FOR HOSPITALS

1. Use at least two patient identifiers when providing care, treatment, and services.
2. Eliminate transfusion errors related to patient misidentification.
3. Report critical results of tests and diagnostics procedures on a timely basis.
4. Label all medications, medication containers, and other solutions on and off the sterile field in perioperative and other procedural settings. *Note*: Medication containers include syringes, medicine cups, and basins.
5. Reduce the likelihood of patient harm associated with the use of anticoagulant therapy.
6. Maintain and communicate accurate patient medication information.
7. Comply with either the current Centers for Disease Control and Prevention (CDC) hand hygiene guidelines or the current World Health Organization (WHO) hand hygiene guidelines.
8. Implement evidence-based practices to prevent health care–associated infections due to multidrug-resistant organisms in acute care hospitals. *Note*: This requirement applies to, but is not limited to, epidemiologically important organisms such as methicillin-resistant *Staphylococcus aureus* (MRSA), *Clostridium difficile* (CDI), Vancomycin-resistant *Enterococci* (VRE), and multidrug-resistant gram-negative bacteria.
9. Implement evidence-based practices to prevent central line–associated blood-stream infections. *Note*: This requirement covers short- and long-term central venous catheters and peripherally inserted central catheter (PICC) lines.

10. Implement evidence-based practices for preventing surgical site infections.
11. Implement evidence-based practices to prevent indwelling catheter-associated urinary tract infections (CAUTI).
12. Identify patients at risk for suicide. *Note*: This requirement applies only to psychiatric hospitals and patients being treated for emotional or behavioral disorders in general hospitals.
13. Conduct a preprocedure verification process.
14. Mark the procedure site.
15. A time out is performed before the procedure.

Joint Commission staff are able medical investigators, and Chassin is a capable chief. The problem is that the Commission is not the right agency to lead the fight against errors. For one thing, the Joint Commission is over-matched by the sheer size of the problem. It has a few hundred staff to inspect thousands of hospitals. Accreditation only occurs on a three-year cycle after a limited number of visits.

The Commission's core mission is state and national accreditations—the assurance of medical competency and not the rooting out of errors and doing justice. Its focus is problem-solving whether in terms of a mistake or not following best practices. Once the correction is made, the Joint Commission moves on and grants accreditation in keeping with the financial realities of health care and the needs of its stakeholders, including the hospitals that pay for its services.

The fourth deemer, the Accreditation Council of Graduate Medical Education (ACGME) has no daily role in error correction or reporting. Nevertheless, the agency stopped a flood of fatigue errors in 2003 by banning overnight call shifts and work weeks exceeding 80 hours for residents. Because the ACGME has the power to shut down residency programs, and because the residents perform much of hospitals' work at bargain rates, the agency is taken seriously.

In the wake of *Too Err is Human*, the epic study of medical mistakes by the Institute of Medicine, Congress began passing legislation. The Healthcare Research and Quality Act of 1999 required the Agency for Healthcare Research and Quality to build "private-public partnerships" to identify causes of preventable errors and patient injury and develop and disseminate strategies to reduce them. In 2005, President George W. Bush signed the Patient Safety and Quality Improvement Act (PSQIA). It authorized the creation of Patient Safety Organizations (PSOs) to gather information on errors and outcomes, perform analysis, and detect patterns of risk and harm.

PSOs are highly diverse. Today there are 76 of them across the country. They include private vendors like General Electric, state hospital associations, profit and non-profit provider networks, and even medical malpractice insurance carriers. Under the PSQIA, PSOs handle "patient safety work product" with "privilege," a wide zone of confidentiality carefully constructed to keep this information out of malpractice litigation. Typically PSOs support websites that present selected cases without noting the names of doctors, patients, or hospitals.

Some that I have read have the feel of mini-studies containing technical language probably beyond the grasp of most laymen. For instance, in one tableau, an apparently healthy older man appeared for a physical by a third-year resident who ordered a prostate-specific antigen (PSA) test. After the resident graduated and left the office, the PSA came back with an elevated score signifying a possible malignancy, but it went unread. An unspecified number of months later the man returned to the office with back pain that turned out to be metastatic prostate cancer. Moral: oversight requires checking lab results ordered by departed doctors. Nothing in the PSO squib indicates whether the cancer victim was told of the error, took action, lived, or died, or even if the adverse event was tallied in a state's reporting system or by Medicare. PSOs' impact on safety is unclear.

In 2014, after one death in America, President Obama appointed an "Ebola Czar" to steer the national response to fear of that scourge. In response to medical errors that claim a quarter million lives annually, we have no leader, little funding, and an alphabet soup of acronyms for public and private actors at the state, local, and federal levels, all doing their own things while gathering, analyzing, censoring, and obscuring information.

In a follow-up analysis of its trenchant study "Hospital Incident Reporting Systems Do Not Capture Most Patient Harm," the DHHS Inspector General made some worrisome points. Of the twenty-six state-reporting systems assessed, most required only a "subset" of events to be reported, usually just fatal or disabling errors and outbreaks of infection. Overall, hospitals were reporting only 1 percent of incidents that Medicare considers adverse events. Moreover, "to date, no Federal standards require States to operate adverse event reporting systems."

Considering the oceans of CMS money that pour into providers, and the fact that 27 percent of Medicare beneficiaries experienced either "serious" incidents "resulting in prolonged hospitalization, permanent disability, life sustaining intervention, or death" or temporary events "requiring intervention but not resulting in lasting harm," and given the extraordinary and tragic difficulties caused by medical errors, the extensive learning opportunities triggered by reporting, and the hefty costs borne by the taxpayer, it would seem to be a no-brainer for Washington to require full-scale reporting from hospitals in exchange for Medicare and Medicaid dollars.

Obviously, the anti-regulatory pushback from the hospitals could be extensive. Some resistance also would come from doctors and nurses asserting that wider reporting would cut into treatment time, a questionable argument since errors inevitably cause additional treatment. Even sturdy defenders of patient safety like Robert Wachter favor smaller reporting systems like Minnesota's that focus on horrendous "never events" and produce "manageable" annual numbers of errors (in the hundreds) for analysis. Somewhat contradictorily, Wachter and other reformers see commercial flight with its sterling and rapid decrease in accidents—a tenfold drop in deaths within a generation—as a model for health care. An acknowledged cause of that industry's safety success is the FAA's Aviation Safety Reporting System (ASRS) which requires mandatory reporting of all accidents, miscues, misdeeds, and near misses as well as crashes whether fatal or not, in all about 35,000 items per year. ASRS gives event reporters strict confidentiality, investigates promptly on a priority basis, has authority to ground planes, close airports, and look for patterns in order to correct product, mechanical, and crew deficiencies.

Wachter points out that the U.S. health-care system could produce 35,000 reports per day and that such a torrent of information would negate any real analysis and render teachable moments too voluminous, but this somewhat misses the point—which is that reporting itself reduces serious errors.

Probably the most puzzling and intriguing part of the Inspector General's depressing study on the paucity of reporting involved Pennsylvania. Fully 55 percent of the incidents reported came from that single state. Why?

In 2004, Pennsylvania became the first and only state to implement mandatory reporting of serious events and incidents in health care, including near misses. In the ensuing decade no other state has adopted full-scale mandatory reporting. Operated by an independent agency called the Pennsylvania Patient Safety Authority, the mandatory Pennsylvania Patient Safety Reporting System covers all hospitals, nursing homes, ambulatory surgical units, birthing centers, and abortion clinics with regard to nine event categories:

1. Medication errors
2. Adverse drug reaction
3. Equipment, supplies, or devices (malfunctions, errors, or failures)

4. Falls
5. Errors related to procedures, treatments, or tests
6. Complications of procedures, treatments, or tests
7. Transfusions
8. Skin Integrity
9. Other, miscellaneous

Reports can be anonymous and are "non-discoverable," which means that they cannot be used in civil (malpractice) litigation. The system is funded by assessments on hospitals and other health-care facilities, and amounts to a tax on lucrative institutions whose "charity" status ordinarily allows them to drain public services without paying for them.

The Pennsylvania system specifies mandatory reporting of every "Serious Event, Incident, and Infrastructure Failure." A Serious Event leads "to death or compromises patient safety and results in an unanticipated injury requiring the delivery of additional health-care services to a patient." Incidents are situations that "could have injured the patient but did not cause an unanticipated injury." Infrastructure Failures pass directly through the Patient Safety Authority to the State Health Department for enforcement and possible prosecution. Relatively rare, they include such crises as *Legionella* outbreaks from contaminated air-conditioning, or surgical fires—horrific eruptions that actually can ignite inside a patient's body—caused by oxygen, lasers, or electrical cautery.

The Pennsylvania System's budget is small—between $5 and 6 million per year—but it amounts to a big bang for the buck since reporting has become virtually universal. The reason probably is because the law makes clear that if the subsequent investigation of an event shows that providers should have reported it but did not, their state licenses to practice medicine or nursing can be lifted. Surprisingly, but probably for the same reason, reporters rarely have resorted to anonymity. In nine years there have been two million reports, but less than a handful have been nameless.

As doctors, nurses, and technicians have come to comprehend what constitute incidents and events (something not well understood in much of the rest of the country, as the DHHS Inspector General wrote) the overall number of items observed and reported has risen somewhat. This does not mean that there were more medical errors—just more were detected. But the greatest impact of the system is that the aggregate data revealed that serious events fell by 12 percent in five years from 8,270 in 2009 to 7,543 in 2013.

In essence, Pennsylvania medicine followed New York cardiac reporting and federal aviation in showing that wide-spread mandatory reporting brought down harmful events. In terms of reducing serious medical errors and plane crashes, rigorous counting helps make it happen, and that includes logging near misses. Of course, this accords with human nature. If you seriously want to lose or maintain weight, get on the scale every day. It is unlikely you will see a big gain.

In addition to decreasing serious events, the decade of Pennsylvania's system of mandatory reporting has reduced Stage III and IV pressure ulcers by 5 percent, wrong-site surgeries by 13 percent, and blood clots by 42 percent.

Patients and their advocates should ask whether their hospital has mandatory recording and reporting of adverse events and errors to a public authority. Citizens should lobby their state governments to implement reporting of all serious events, incidents, and near misses.

Currently, two national frameworks also impact oversight of health care: the courts (malpractice) and Medicare (bouncebacks). The *raison d'etre* of malpractice, also known as medical negligence, is to compensate victims of health-care harms. With the media glare on medical errors in the late twentieth century came a "malpractice boom." Much loathed by physicians and insurance companies, it produced about 15,000 annual cases at its peak. More recently the number has descended to about 9,500.

In *To Err is Human*, the Institute of Medicine conservatively estimated that 1 out of 100 hospital patients experienced a serious preventable injury and only 1.5 percent of those filed a malpractice suit. Even the most overt and blatant of screw-ups—operations performed on wrong sites or patients—seldom led to cases, since only 21.5 percent of these victims sued. As Tom Baker, a professor at the University of Pennsylvania Law School and scholar of malpractice put it, "We have an epidemic of medical malpractice, not of malpractice law suits."

Glamorized by Hollywood, "runaway jury" (the title of a John Grisham novel and film) awards are rarities rather than norms. Surveys of state malpractice verdicts and settlements show that they average between $100,000 and $200,000.

The heyday of malpractice and malpractice fears produced positive and negative changes in medicine. Record keeping by doctors and nurses vastly improved as did ways to separate lookalike drugs. Anesthesiologists began continuously monitoring oxygen levels of patients during surgery, which prevented many deaths. In general, these specialists above others tried to learn from litigation.

During the 1970s, the American Society of Anesthesiologists implemented a rigorous profession-wide "closed claims project" to analyze, publicize, and derive better priorities from errors that arose in lawsuits. Before the project, anesthesiology was among the most dangerous and sued specialties with 1 in 10,000 patients dying on the table. 7.9 percent of all malpractice claims were anesthesiology-based. Afterwards the death rate fell to 1 in 200,000, the percentage of negligence claims slipped to 3.8 percent, and insurance premiums dropped.

Malpractice also helped to identify horrible physicians—the 6 percent of doctors responsible for nearly 60 percent of all medical negligence. While courts shine a light on these "bad apples" they seldom endure sanctions from state licensing boards. Two-thirds of those who had ten or more malpractice claims received no discipline and continued practicing (and malpracticing).

Because the code of litigation is silence, these errors usually are not probed in hospital grand rounds, morbidity and mortality conferences, or disciplinary proceedings sometimes known as peer reviews. Since 1990, most disciplinary actions, like negligent events leading to compensation, must be revealed to the National Practitioner's Data Bank (NPDB). Doctors understandably want to avoid these official blots if possible. The American Medical Association even puts out a pamphlet entitled "How to Evade a Report to the NPDB" with timely tips like getting a suspension limited to twenty-nine days since thirty or more must be recorded.

Since 1990 almost half of U.S. hospitals have failed to report even a single disciplinary action to the NPDB. Half of physicians also admit that they see and fail to report incompetence. So Dr. HODAD and other miscreants remain safe, while their patients suffer.

Doctors who make mistakes not rising to the level of malpractice, or whose patients experience poor low frequency outcomes, sometimes get sued resulting in a grueling four- to five-year experience for practitioners and patients. To avoid lawsuits, physicians practice "defensive medicine." They conduct unnecessary tests and procedures, make shotgun diagnoses to rule out even the remotest causes of symptoms, and call in unnecessary specialists.

Some studies have shown that defensive medicine adds $50 to 60 billion to the national health bill. The George W. Bush administration argued that the tag price could be over $100 billion, a claim the Congressional Budget Office failed to support because some of this deluxe "try-everything" approach is based on revenue production, a phenomenon cynically known as "using the patient as an ATM" rather than actual fear of litigation. Regardless, defensive medicine manifests itself in real ways including calling for more Caesarean sections than necessary, painful breast biopsies, rampant CT scanning with attendant over-radiation in emergency rooms, and expanded hospital stays that cannot be medically justified. Surveys show that over 90 percent of doctors have practiced defensive medicine at some point in their careers.

The health care and insurance industries also pushed back against medical malpractice with a spate of legal measures called tort reform. These began in California in the 1980s with caps on non-economic emotional distress damages and spread to forty states. The caps range from $250,000 to $500,000 and often make it unrealistic for injured children, the elderly, or others without lost earnings to prosecute claims. Other measures include shortening statutes of limitations to as little as a year, blocking punitive damages, letting juries deduct other forms of payment like automobile and workers' compensation insurance, limiting potential rewards by substituting "fair share" rules for joint and several liability exposure for each actor in the chain of causation, making plaintiffs retain and pay experts when they file the case, and preventing victims from introducing apologies from doctors and nurses into evidence, a practice not followed in other types of law. In many jurisdictions, defendants win over 90 percent of malpractice verdicts.

Why are so many cases lost, and so few victims compensated? Recently I spoke with Alan Perer, a leading plaintiff's malpractice attorney who handled a "dizzy stroke" death case in 2014. Three years before, his client—an otherwise healthy 56-year-old husband and father of two—arrived by ambulance at the emergency room of a small suburban hospital that was a member of a well-regarded regional health system. The man's symptoms included sweating, nausea, vomiting, vertigo, and a stabbing occipital (back of the head) headache. The emergency physicians knew that their mission was to rule out or identify a cebrovascular attack—in plain terms, a stroke.

With ischemic (blockage) stokes, patients often can be cured if they receive an intravenous thrombolytic (clot busting) agent called Tissue Plasminogen Activator (TPA) that must flow within three hours (ideally 90 minutes) of onset. The ER doctors sent the patient for a CT scan. CT is far less expensive than MRI, but MRIs better define ischemic strokes in the cerebellar arterial network in the back of the brain. Probably because they were not trained to do so, the doctors failed to perform the rapid eye movement observations promoted by the Newman-Toker team at Johns Hopkins which are cost-free and likely as accurate as MRIs.

The regional health system also had advertised that it provided "telestroke" protection. In other words, a patient who presented with symptoms at an outlying hospital could be televised in real time to a neurologist trained to detect rapid eye movements. Remarkably, the suburban doctors failed to avail themselves of this service. The CT scan came back normal and the physicians ruled out giving TPA.

The patient's erosion continued. His blood pressure spiked with severe back of the head pain and his eyes visibly diverted to the right. Five hours after admission, an MRI finally was performed that revealed ischemic stroke but it was too late for TPA. With substantial swelling and brain damage, the patient was helicoptered to the health system's flagship hospital, where he underwent a series of cranial surgeries and decompressions, suffered subsequent strokes, and died in two weeks. The deceased had been the financial mainstay of his family. Although money could not replace him, the economic losses ran into the millions.

Fundamentally not about mistakes or errors, malpractice is meant to compensate victims and families when the treatment, which need not be ideal, is proven to have sunk below the "standard of care." The trial turned into a duel of experts with those for the doctors and hospital inveighing successfully that the initial

CT scan met the professional standard while the family's doctor claimed that other more reliable methods would have caught the clot, triggered TPA in time, and saved the man. The jury's deliberations were short. The defendants were not liable, the family was not compensated, and no information from the case went into NPDB or any data repository from which better practices could be discerned and taught. Afterwards, unprevailing attorney Perer lamented the limits of the malpractice system including that "sometimes in order to win, defendants depress the standard of care instead of standing up for best practices."

Even in the minority of situations when medically injured people receive compensation through the malpractice process, legal and overhead costs grab approximately 60 percent of payouts. Since the late twentieth century an alternative called "health courts" has drawn policy makers' attention without making much political headway.

Somewhat like the workers' compensation non-jury system that pays employees set amounts for defined harms or death, health courts now exist in Denmark, Finland, Norway, Sweden, and New Zealand. Some health courts apply a no-fault standard. Sweden and Denmark use an "availability" test such that if a medically appropriate practice or treatment could have prevented the harm, then the patient receives payment. Barriers to admission to the system for victims are fairly low: ten days of additional treatment or thirty days off work typically suffice. Any long-term or permanent injury qualifies. Proceedings are usually completed within six to nine months of the accident. Lawyers are optional. Victims often choose doctors or other care workers as their advocates. The judicial panel of mainly physicians retains neutral experts at no expense to the parties. Administrative expenses run to about 17 percent. The majority of victims are compensated. Payouts are low by U.S. standards, usually in five figures, and there are overall caps on awards. The highest is $1.7 million in Denmark. Data from health-court cases is processed by national agencies in order to establish trends and teach prevention.

Health courts are popular in their societies, but meet resistance in the U.S. especially over the low compensation levels that are driven by the reality that those countries provide lifetime free universal single-payer health care. Essentially that means that the foreign awards unlike ours do not need to cover victims' future (even lifetime) care, drugs, and rehabilitation. No one including advocates believes that U.S. health courts would pay at the low levels of New Zealand or Scandinavia given the realities of our largely pay-as-you-go partial-coverage health-care system, but seven and eight figure judgments would be rare.

During the past century, special courts became a part of the American legal landscape including business tribunals like the Delaware Court of Chanery, the United States Tax Court, and the Federal Court of Claims. There has been some spread into health-related areas including Social Security Disability administrative tribunals, and a neutral quasi-court in the Department of Health and Human Services for childhood vaccine injuries.

In the wake of the terror attacks of September 11, 2001, Congress enabled funds to provide no-fault awards to victims in the air and on the ground. In a 1980s insurance crisis when obstetricians had trouble getting coverage, Florida and Virginia started limited no-fault nonjury health courts to compensate families when children suffered neurological injuries during birth. These were "opt out" systems not vulnerable to constitutional challenges since families could chose to put their claims in malpractice courts with juries, higher burdens of proof, and smaller opportunities to win, but potentially larger awards. More recently, Kaiser Permanente, the nation's largest HMO, gave patients the opportunity to arbitrate malpractice claims and more than six million members have signed up in the hope of prompt, fair, likely awards (albeit at lower rates than a jury could award) if they ever suffer medical injuries.

As with all aspects of the malpractice debate, health courts are polarizing. Democrats and trial lawyers react vociferously and unrealistically against these Scandinavian safety net vehicles of widespread compensation for victims. Republicans have been just as irrational, reportedly pushing back hard during Affordable Care Act debates against proposed reforms that would have freed doctors from liability by giving them flat-out immunity from injury claims when they followed approved best practices guidelines or checklists.

Another measure much in the interest of providers and insurance carriers would have compensated victims through the Federal Tort Claims Act. Covered doctors nominally would have to become partial federal employees. Already they are multiply employed by their practice groups, universities, hospitals, HMOs, and professional corporations. The addition of the federal employment slice simply would have recognized the reality that they also are paid in large part by the feds including through Medicare, Medicaid, and and military insurance. Predictably the plan was turned down as too "socialistic."

Somehow health courts survived in principle in the ACA. Tucked into an obscure corner of the legislation is $50 million for development of state projects. These hopefully will turn into additional alternatives to malpractice tribunals, where victims will gain speedy justice including a realistic standard of fault (or no fault) leading to fair compensation with limited overhead. Further, data from medical accidents will be allowed to flow freely and sufficiently into a national system of oversight and analysis.

Though it was not his intent, President George W. Bush sparked such a system when he signed the Deficit Reduction Act (DRA) of 2005. At the time, fear loomed large that Medicare would go belly-up and that health-care costs would bankrupt older Americans. The Congressional Budget Office predicted that as a percentage of Gross Domestic Product, health care would rise from 16 percent in 2007 to 25 percent in 2025 and to 49 percent in 2082.

Since poor quality had been identified by the Institute of Medicine as a driver of inflated costs, the DRA mandated CMS to choose "at least two hospital acquired conditions or errors for which it no longer would pay." After consulting with the Centers for Disease Control and Prevention, CMS came up with a list of eleven "no pay" items.

1. Object inadvertently left in after surgery
2. Air embolism
3. Blood incompatibility
4. Catheter associated urinary tract infection
5. Pressure ulcer (decubitus ulcer)
6. Vascular catheter associated infection
7. Surgical site infection—Mediastinitis (infection in the chest)—after coronary artery bypass graft surgery
8. Certain types of falls and traumas
9. Surgical site infections following certain elective procedures, including certain orthopedic surgeries, and bariatric surgery for obesity
10. Certain manifestations of poor control of blood sugar levels
11. Deep vein thrombosis or pulmonary embolism following total knee replacement and hip replacement procedures.

In 2007, CMS added Present On Admission (POA) information to the software that hospitals must use when submitting claims to Medicare. So, if any of the eleven errors and conditions on the no-pay list were not charted when the patient was admitted, CMS would refuse to fund them since they were "hospital acquired." Now known as "P4P" (pay for performance) the quality-oriented system saves taxpayers about $60 million annually and forces providers to stem errors or eat their related costs.

The Affordable Care Act also allowed CMS to punish unplanned readmissions within thirty days after discharge. Presumed errors if unplanned, these "bounce-backs" cost the taxpayers over $17 billion per year and result from confusing discharge, medication, and therapy instructions, poor communication among providers, and lack-of-compliance errors by patients. CMS recoups about $300 million per year from bounce-back penalties that critics say fall hardest on hospitals that treat the poor and medically illiterate. Regardless, the program has had overwhelmingly positive effects including halting a chronic racket that occurred when hospitals that received set amounts from CMS for patients' stays for various treatments discharged people early in order to maximize profits.

To avoid bounce-backs and resulting fines, hospitals increasingly send visiting nurses to patients' homes to help them with drugs, wound care, and keeping appointments. Better discharge planning now involves screening patients to determine who will need more help before and after going home. Likely to bounce-back people include those in poor health, the depressed, and those taking five or more medications.

The Centers for Medicare & Medicaid Services is a sprawling agency comprising 4 percent of GDP with over half a trillion dollars in outlays per year. It has proven efficient and popular: 72 percent of Americans favor Medicare including 87 percent of those over 65. 64 percent support Medicaid, 71 percent in households making $40 thousand or less. Since passage of the ACA in 2010, the agency also runs a program that gives bonuses or penalties to hospitals on other quality measures. These incentives assess how quickly patients having heart attacks receive angioplasties (known as "door to balloon" time) in addition to Medicare patient ratings on how well doctors and nurses communicated with them during their hospital stays.

Especially while external reporting of medical errors to accreditors and governmental agencies remains fragmentary, internal oversight at provider institutions should be as strong as possible. Teamwork remains critical to building a safety culture. Every doctor and nurse should have the opportunity to receive full information, be able to scrutinize the contributions of others, and be encouraged to speak up when anything goes wrong. Everyone on the team literally should be on the same page, whether it is a checklist for a catheter, surgical procedure, infection control, or particularly an unforeseen emergency outcome, which is an especially difficult contingency for teams including members who rarely work together in large health-care organizations.

Chesley "Sully" Sullenberger, the pilot of the U.S. Airways passenger jet that landed without loss of life on the Hudson River in 2009, regards that outcome as a team effort with his crew, and especially with co-pilot Jeff Skiles whom he barely knew. Moreover, the airline never had practiced water landings, and there was not enough data on these events to train for them on flight simulators. Thus, teams had engaged only in "a theoretical class-room discussion" of water landings. But all were trained to absorb and share data in manageable bites during a crisis. While a pilot, Sullenberger participated in accident investigations. Since retirement he has shared his expertise with other high-risk industries including health care, which he finds inferior to aviation due to barriers on information flow:

> What would it take in medicine? I can tell you that if we, as airline pilots, operated in a system as fragmented, as imperfect as you do, we'd have similar outcomes. If our airplanes were designed like some ICU's and OR's in which there was insufficient integration—in which they weren't sufficiently connected—in which information was not appropriately shared—we couldn't operate the way we do.

Information must be palatable and manageable especially in a crisis. Recipients cannot feel like they are pulling teeth or trying to drink from a fire hose.

Eagerly awaited and deeply encouraging, a study on "Changes in Medical Errors After Implementation of a Hand-off

Program" appeared in the *New England Journal of Medicine* on November 6, 2014. Hand-offs of patient responsibility and information between residents as shifts change long has been a source of serious medical errors. Miscommunications during these critical transitions contribute to two-thirds of sentinel events (those that cause death or serious injury) according to the Joint Commission. Plus, due to the worthy reforms of limiting residents' duty hours (and errors from fatigue), hand-offs have increased and so have fears that communication errors have grown accordingly.

The *NEJM* study, which sought to reduce errors from hand-offs, occurred at nine hospitals in the U.S. and Canada between January 2011 and May 2013. Stimulated by a new Accreditation Council for Graduate Medical Education requirement for residency programs to enhance training and monitor the quality of hand-offs, the study tested the safety of a bundled information protocol called I-Pass. Developed at Boston Children's Hospital, one of the participating institutions, it spread to the other eight. A mnemonic, I-Pass stands for "illness severity, patient summary, action list, situation awareness and contingency planning, and synthesis or read back."

A total of 875 residents participated. For the first six months of the study, they were untrained on I-Pass, and conducted hand-offs according to their usual practices. Then they received a period of training so they could convey and receive I-Pass information both orally and in writing through the bundle's software.

In all, the residents followed a total of 10,740 pediatric patients, 5,516 during the "pre-intervention" (before training) period and 5,224 post-intervention. The cases were vetted for the occurrence of medical errors. The pediatric patients in both periods of the study were quite similar in terms of race, sex, public insurance, complexity of treatment, and length of stay. The amount of time residents spent at bedside, with families, and at computers also stayed constant. The oral hand-offs were recorded on video before and after intervention, and these also did not change significantly in duration: 2.4 minutes (before), 2.5 minutes (after).

In all, the rate of medical errors declined by 23 percent between the pre- and post-intervention periods. Preventable adverse advents to the pediatric patients actually decreased by 30 percent. Non-preventable adverse events remained virtually constant during both periods, a good sign of the experiment's validity. The I-Pass results indicate that even in the trenches of high-volume care, free-flowing intelligently shaped information with oversight and monitoring makes patients safer. This principle has also been vindicated in private practice.

In 2010, the *American Journal of Gastroenterology* published "The Impact of Video Recording on the Quality of Colonoscopy Performance: A Pilot Study," an intriguing experiment where physicians were tricked into revealing their true deficient practices and then into improving them. Designed by Douglas Rex, a renowned gastroenterologist at the University of Indiana, it focused on colonoscopies by seven active doctors in Indianapolis.

With the collusion of nurses, these physicians were told falsely that their procedures were not being digitally video-recorded through their colonoscopes. For subsequent colonoscopies, they were told truthfully that their work would be recorded and evaluated, including on the time allotted and quality of the procedure. Each of the physicians recorded seven "pre-awareness" and seven "post-awareness" procedures for a total of 98 videos.

Often difficult and disturbing for patients, colonoscopies can discover colorectal cancers called adenomas as well as precancerous polyps. But the procedures are "operator dependent" and when performed poorly fail to detect malignancies that can metastasize and become fatal. So-called "miss rates" rise when doctors take shortcuts. With proper use of the colonoscope there is a rigorous examination of folds, full luminal distention (keeping the scope's walls spread apart), careful cleaning of obscuring surface debris, and adequate time spent on the test, generally seven or eight minutes.

Dr. Rex and his team scored the quality of the pre-aware and post-aware colonoscopies from 1 to 5 for all the physicians. They found that quality dipped dangerously when operators lacked awareness of scrutiny but jumped when doctors knew they would face review.

Subsequently, the seven Indiana gastroenterologists started video-recording all colonoscopies and quality remained high. Other departments followed suit. The Rex group began offering patients their internal videos on DVDs and found that 81 percent wanted them. Interest peaked among those with personal or family histories of cancer, and others concerned about "miss rates." All could take the valuable digital recording to another physician for a second opinion, or use it for comparison with a later test. They were safer.

Patients and their advocates should request that their surgeries and internal procedures be video recorded (if safe and practical) and further ask to obtain copies. In general, cameras and other forms of oversight deter low-quality unsafe behaviors among providers ranging from hand-hygiene avoidance to surgical shortcuts.

■

We cannot know what happened to the pediatric residents who made errors during the first round of the I-Pass study, or to the video-recorded gastroenterologists unaware that their low-quality procedures were being recorded, much less to their patients who may or may not have received their DVDs and could have gotten new colonoscopies.

What is supposed to happen following errors in our fragmented, accreditory and loosely regulated system? How are errors supposed to be processed at least at the local institutional level?

The Joint Commission requires accredited hospitals to hold a "root cause analysis" after every sentinel event. Called RCAs, these structured reviews may or may not actually take place. If they do probably depends upon whether the institution has a safety culture backed by management. Also, RCAs are required under some states' laws.

The RCA process varies widely across and even inside institutions. A major divider is confidentiality driven by fear of "medicolegal risk." In the past, RCAs generally did not disclose errors or causes of harm to patients for fear they would sue.

The modern trend involves full disclosure "to the patient and family that an unanticipated event has occurred," said T. Michael White, M.D., an internist who served as a vice president/chief medical officer for a health-care system in Maryland and for two Pennsylvania hospitals with responsibility for quality and patient safety, and an inspector for both the Joint Commission and ACGME. Now a consultant to hospitals on safety, White recommends that local leadership assign a patient advocate to gain the error victim's and family's insight into the accident, provide feedback to them on the investigation, and be their voice at the RCA. Management also appoints an interdisciplinary team to find the source of the lapse, whether a weak staffing ratio, communications glitch, equipment failure, or otherwise. Standing RCAs such as at the University of California at San Francisco usually meet once a week for about two hours and no session concludes without a "clear action plan and assigned responsibilities," according to Robert Wachter.

The needs of the traumatized or injured patients also are met, including referrals to necessary support services. Moreover, payment of a settlement often is discussed at this early juncture, which marks a sea charge for a profession that historically has been inclined to duck the issue for years or forever. As a rule, patients and their advocates should request that any mistakes in treatment be reported to them and referred for root cause analysis.

"Secondary victims"—the doctors and nurses involved in errors—likewise can receive care, support, therapy, and help with making their presentations in situations that can be emotionally devastating. While the RCA process looks for human error, it attempts not to castigate providers but to find correctable systems errors. RCA fundamentally is not a discipline process often known as "peer review" whose contents mainly are confidential, privileged, and excludable from malpractice cases.

Another key point about RCAs is that they "triage"—overwhelmingly focusing on the gravest accidents in the brief time allotted—which means that less damaging cases and near misses may receive little or no attention from the group.

■

In terms of preventing medical errors, probably nothing is as important to hospitals as creating a safety culture. This is not an easy task given other priorities like assembling a competent staff, delivering treatment, and budgeting. How does management put safety first? To some extent, safety can be incorporated into training, checklists, reporting, and surveillance, but physicians come and go in hospitals. With the exceptions of hospitalists and residents, they perform their surgeries, procedures, make rounds, and return to their practices. Generally they do their own thing according to their own standards, credentials, and experience, and raise few hints of problems. "Doctors don't report errors," said White. "Nurses do," echoing the finding of the DHHS Inspector General.

As a hospital chief medical and and quality officer, White distributed scholarship on safety and ramped up prevention efforts in advance of Joint Commission site reviews. "I could say we must do this or that because of the Joint Commission. I loved it when they were coming. I could move mountains." But the Commission came only once every three years and everyone on staff knew that it was basically impossible for a hospital to be decertified.

White became a convener and believer in root cause analysis, and his hospitals had standing weekly triaged sessions for sentinel errors. As the leader, he appointed investigators, derived information from staff and patients involved, and ultimately held a prophylactic session that would find the reason for a mistake as well as take steps to prevent it from cropping up again. In his training paper "Advancing Health Care Value through Cause Analysis", White describes how a theoretical RCA in a 200-bed suburban hospital (like the one where a patient's dizzy stroke went undetected) could be utilized to identify the cause of an apparently healthy young man becoming unresponsive and failing to breathe following a knee replacement.

The model RCA revealed that the patient was not screened adequately for sleep apnea, putting him at risk for narcotic-induced respiratory failure. Inadequate training and communications of admitting staff and anesthesiologists were found to be factors. Other potential factors such as fatigue, demographic inequality, and lack of professionalism were ruled out. An RCA in such a case could be transformative and prevent such an adverse event from ever happening again. "If I only had one tool to change the culture of an organization it would be root cause analysis," said White, who spent a four-decade career focused on improving patient safety.

It makes sense for patients and their advocates to ask hospitals and departments how many root cause analyses they have held in a year. If the providers say "zero" or "only a few," that speaks poorly for safety, because there is no shortage of sentinel errors in most emergency and patient settings. Not analyzing these problems through RCAs is to minimize them, avoid learning and prevention, and flout the Joint Commission's core obligation as well.

Sometimes with the cooperation of physicians involved, RCA errors can become the subject of a morbidity and mortality (M&M) conference, a type of grand round where a case is dissected academically to the doctors in a department and perhaps to the hospital at large.

While extremely difficult, heartbreaking, and grim, it also makes sense for families and advocates to seek autopsies when patients die in treatment. Post-mortems show that about a quarter of the deceased experienced errors in hospitals. Since Semmelweis' time it has been known that autopsies are a place to look for answers to fatal problems. Families, advocates, and providers sometimes can prevent similar losses to others by using these exercises to recover explanations from the dead.

■

Reporting and oversight of medical errors remains uneven and deficient, which in some ways is surprising given the enormous deference—some would say lip service—that health care pays to the aviation and nuclear industries. While medicine has studied and absorbed some of their teamwork, checklist, and emergency drill practices, it has been slow to adopt mandatory disclosure to agencies such as occurs with the Federal Aviation Administration and Nuclear Regulatory Commission that are credited with nearly eliminating major errors like crashes and meltdowns. A big part of some of their industries' success involves compulsory error reporting internally and externally to oversight agencies. Parenthetically, when units of the Veterans Administration surprisingly in 2014 were revealed to have committed fraud, which resulted in the resignation of VA Secretary Eric Shinseki, it became apparent that there was no way for patients and their families to complain beyond and outside their VA hospitals to an oversight agency.

Assuming there should be an oversight layer beyond the particular hospitals or clinics to whom all serious errors and near misses could be reported as in Pennsylvania, who would do it? Cash strapped and budget-bound, the states will not. Pennsylvania is a promising aberration, and even it lacks the swift enforcement mechanism that Pronovost has advocated for shutting down a hospital committing fatal errors as surely as a mine is closed following a deadly explosion.

Strong federal precedents for oversight compliance systems exist in other key areas of interstate commerce crucial to national safety and values. It is hard to imagine a field that spreads beyond state borders more than health care, which attracts physicians, patients, pharmaceuticals, and equipment from everywhere. The National Highway Transportation Safety Administration gathers and studies all complaints of automotive defects. The same is true for the U.S. Department of Justice and Equal Employment Opportunities Commission regarding alleged civil rights violations, and the Federal Trade Commission and Securities Exchange Commission, which field complaints of attacks on free enterprise including price fixing, monopolies, and stock and bond frauds.

But there are so many medical errors in the United States, probably upwards of ten million each year. The scale of magnitude dwarfs the responsibilities of agencies concerned with cars, planes, and civil rights.

What would be the lead federal agency for health care? Doctors and nurses concerned with safety and not hostile to such regulation seem to favor the Agency for Healthcare Research Quality (AHRQ) or Central Medicare & Medicaid Services for this role. AHRQ (pronounced "arc") has done good work in terms of funding error studies and publishing the annual National Healthcare Quality Report. But AHRQ is small, lacks a connection to the American public, is politically weak, and shies away from the key issue of sizing the error problem that in turn relates to wider issues of funding and enforcement.

In 2014 AHRQ still adhered to the 1999 Institute of Medicine estimate of 44,000 to 98,000 deaths, which has been superseded by global trigger tool studies. Persistent minimization reduces the responsibility of health care for this man-made epidemic constituting our third largest source of death, and is reminiscent of the medical apologists in 1999 who claimed that the IOM figure was wildly inflated.

CMS however is a huge powerful agency with strong public approval and a burgeoning cost-effective anti-error mission based on bounce-backs. Through its Inspector General analysis, CMS well knows the scope of damage. About one in four hospitalized Medicare patients suffers harm, including more than 180,000 deaths per year, a figure that signals a substantial disconnect with AHRQ's estimated use of the IOM figure of fewer than 100,000 (for all Americans, not just Medicare recipients).

Plus, it wound not be a great stretch for CMS's error protection to extend to more Americans who are not simply victims of bounce-backs and from Medicare's eleven-item no-pay list. Two other well-regarded lists have been used to compute errors. The first is AHRQ's Patient Safety Indicator (PSIs). Ironically, when global triggers are applied to PSIs (which appear below) estimates of national deaths reach a quarter million.

AGENCY FOR HEALTHCARE RESEARCH AND QUALITY'S (AHRQ) PATIENT SAFETY INDICATORS (PSIs)

1. Death in low-mortality diagnosis-related groups
2. Pressure ulcer
3. Death among surgical inpatients with treatable serious complications
4. Foreign body left in during procedure
5. Iatrogenic pneumothorax
6. Central venous catheter-related bloodstream infections
7. Postoperative hip fracture
8. Postoperative hemorrhage or hematoma
9. Postoperative physiologic and metabolic derangements
10. Postoperative respiratory failure
11. Postoperative pulmonary embolism or deep vein thrombosis
12. Postoperative sepsis

13. Postoperative wound dehiscence
14. Accidental puncture or laceration
15. Transfusion reaction
16. Birth Trauma—injury to neonate
17. Obstetric—vaginal delivery with instrument
18. Obstetric—vaginal delivery without instrument

To safety-oriented members of the medical profession, probably the most highly regarded roster of errors (perhaps because it focuses on decidedly grave incidents) is the National Quality Forum's (NQF) twenty-nine item "List of Serious Reportable Events." A non-profit standard-setting entity encompassing over 400 medical and pharmaceutical organizations, NQF emerged from Presidential recommendations following the 1999 Institute of Medicine Report. Sometimes its compilation is called the "never events" list because these harms never should occur in any hospital or clinical environment. The overlaps with the AHRQ list appear in bold type.

THE NATIONAL QUALITY FORUM'S LIST OF SERIOUS REPORTABLE EVENTS

Surgical or invasive procedure events
1. Surgery of other invasive procedure performed on the wrong site
2. Surgery or other invasive procedure performed on the wrong patient
3. Wrong surgical or other invasive procedure performed on a patient
4. Unintended retention of a foreign object in a patient after surgery or other invasive procedure
5. Intraoperative or immediately postoperative death in an ASA Class 1 patient[1]

---

1 An American Society of Anesthesiologists (ASA) Class 1 patient is normally healthy.

Product or device events

6. Patient death or serious injury associated with the use of contaminated drugs, devices, or biologics provided by the health-care setting

7. Patient death or serious injury associated with the use or function of a device in patient care, in which the device is used for functions other than as intended

8. Patient death or serious injury associated with intravascular air embolism that occurs while being cared for in a health-care setting

Patient protection events

9. Discharge or release of a patient/resident of any age, who is unable to make decisions, to other than an authorized person

10. Patient death or serious injury associated with patient elopement (disappearance)

11. Patient suicide, attempted suicide, or self-harm that results in serious injury, while being cared for in a health-care setting

Care management events

12. Patient death or serious injury associated with a medication error (e.g. errors involving the wrong drug, wrong dose, wrong patient, wrong time, wrong preparation, or wrong route of administration)

13. Patient death or serious injury associated with unsafe administration of blood products

14. Maternal death or serious injury associated with labor or delivery in a low-risk pregnancy while being cared for in a health-care setting

15. Death or serious injury of a neonate associated with labor or delivery in a low-risk pregnancy (new in 2011)

16. Patient death or serious injury associated with a fall while being cared for in a health-care setting

17. Any Stage 3, Stage 4, and unstageable pressure ulcers acquired after admission/presentation to a health-care setting
18. Artificial insemination with the wrong donor sperm or wrong egg
19. Patient death or serious injury resulting from the irretrievable loss of an irreplaceable biological specimen (new in 2011)
20. Patient death or serious injury resulting from failure to follow up or communicate laboratory, pathology, or radiology test results (new in 2011)

Environmental events
21. Patient or staff death or serious injury associated with an electric shock in the course of a patient care process in a health-care setting
22. Any incident in which systems designated for oxygen or other gas to be delivered to a patient contain no gas, the wrong gas, or are contaminated by toxic substances
23. Patient or staff death or serious injury associated with a burn incurred from any source in the course of a patient care process in a health-care setting
24. Patient death or serious injury associated with the use of physical restraints or bedrails while being cared for in a health-care setting

Radiologic events
25. Death or serious injury of a patient or staff associated with the introduction of a metallic object into the MRI area

Potential criminal events
26. Any instance of care ordered by or provided by someone impersonating a physician, nurse, pharmacist, or other licensed health-care provider

27. Abduction of a patient/resident of any age
28. Sexual abuse/assault on a patient or staff member within or on the grounds of a health-care setting
29. Death or serious injury of a patient or staff member resulting from a physical assault (i.e. battery) that occurs within or on the grounds of a health-care setting

The sum of the AHRQ and NQF would be a highly-protective combined range of forty-two reportable errors. CMS then automatically could levy a fine for each error, collecting funds to pay for Medicare and Medicaid patients' treatments, strengthen its bottom line, and give hospitals, nursing homes, and other providers a major financial incentive to stop hurting people. Errors involving grave injury, death, or particularly disturbing features could spur further investigations.

Much of the system largely could be automated as with bounce-backs. There could be an appeal process to the Department of Health and Human Services and then if necessary into court. Also, a category could exist for "near misses" that would not need to be fined. Simply reporting them and if necessary investigating them likely would lead to declines in serious errors. A comprehensive error and near-miss system with oversight is as necessary in health care as it is in aviation and nuclear energy. Hospitalized Americans are no less valuable and are far more endangered than miners, airline passengers, or nuclear plant neighbors.

In some ways, patients already are better positioned to protect themselves than other potential victims of accidents. Unlike say aviation customers most patients actually can see and do certain things to avoid errors. To be sure this ability is limited and many health-care mistakes—whether about medications, infections, or hand-offs—hinge on communications. Many patients do not speak English (about 20 percent) and providers often lack adequate interpreter services. Other patients have a mental or physical inability to participate, or they lack sufficient medical literacy (perhaps 50 percent) to understand their care.

In most complex or long-term cases, it helps for the patients to have an advocate or advisor at their side. Such a person can be a family member or friend. When not available, some hospitals may assign one. Often, says T. Michael White, such advocates are social workers, and they pop up when there has been trouble, say an adverse event, poor outcome, or error. Typically such advocates may work in the same organizational silos as risk managers, which can lead to conflicts if protecting the institution comes into play.

White favors using independent individuals whom he calls Personal Professional Patient Advocates (P3As). Through training or background, they can "understand the complexity of the health-care process," can review the chart, assist in fathoming treatment, participate in family meetings and, when necessary, communicate in a "respectful, efficient, and articulate way to the health-care team." Loyal, semi-retired providers like White, 67, make ideal P3As, and he has played this role for family members, sometimes sparing them aggressive or unnecessary treatments.

Altruistic, well-trained P3As may become more prevalent in the future. In the near term most of us probably will have to wade through the swamps of health care alone or with whatever help we can get from friends, relatives, and primary care physicians, who should be notified as soon as patients enter the hospital. It cannot be taken for granted that the health-care system automatically has included the PCP in the circle of those made aware of an emergency or in-patient treatment. Even when notified it cannot be assumed that all but the most exceptional PCPs suddenly will become day-to-day round-the-clock advocates of the best and safest treatment for patients, especially in hospitals where they do not normally round or have staff privileges.

Still, as White says, medicine "has its own language." So, to the extent possible, it makes sense to have a doctor on the patient's side with limited loyalty to anyone else including the institution, which also cannot be trusted to have a current version of the patient's medical record. Hence, every patient should maintain an updated list of medications, dosages, illnesses, surgeries, allergies, adverse reactions, and treatments. Patients should try to develop positive long-term relations with PCPs who under ideal circumstances could become their care team overseers and coordinators in crises, but this has become more difficult in the specialized and stratified managed-care era.

∎

U.S. medicine favors wealthy, educated, verbal, well-connected people. However, all patients and advocates should attempt oversight of their care in four fundamental ways: monitoring, making friends, speaking up, and teaching back.

Monitoring care: All states and the federal government allow patients to access their medical records. In the pre-internet era that often meant securing paper copies and paying for them. In-patients however could read their charts for free on a clipboard found in the wire basket at the foot of the bed. Electronic data made the situation easier for out-patients, but more difficult for those in hospitals who could not simply reach for the clipboard to see the results of their labs and x-rays, and were not taught or permitted to make the few keystrokes on consoles to open this information. Now patients and their advocates (who may need limited health-care powers of attorney) can log onto electronic records with their phones, laptops, and tablets. Patients also should assure that their PCPs receive all hospital treatment information in real time as it develops. Monitoring means being watchful that staff wash their hands, remove catheters on time, give pills on schedule, and keep IV bags from going dry.

Making friends: That means being friendly with nurses, doctors, and other staff, knowing their names, and getting them to repeat the patient's name at least once a shift. It's a good idea to become familiar with personnel on different shifts, so a patient can ask if Dr. Jones knows that Dr. Smith earlier reduced a drug. Making friends means standing up for decent staff working conditions and asking whether a resident is too fatigued to write an order or insert a line, or if the nursing ratios are inadequate to maintain safe conditions. For instance, in medical and surgical departments nurse-to-patient ratios of higher than 6–7: 1 lead to increased errors. In ICUs, nurses must be much more plentiful. Here, the ratio actually shouldn't be greater than 2: 1 for safety to be maintained.

The mix matters too. Errors rise when Registered Nurses start delivering less than 70 percent of care, and cheaper providers like Licensed Practical Nurses and nurses' aides provide more than 30 percent. Similarly it is unfair to residents to serve as the only overnight doctors. Patients and their advocates should request/insist on a senior attending physician being in the hospital till morning.

Speaking up: Obviously, it is important to be vocal and direct with providers. It is so critical that the Joint Commission has initiated a "Speak-Up Campaign" in its thousands of accredited hospitals to foster safer environments where the voices of patients, families, friends, advisors, and supporters, are not hushed as annoyances but expected to be heard and heeded. The Joint Commission urges patients in its hospitals to "speak-up if you have questions or concerns. If you still do not understand, ask again. It is your body and you have a right to know. "Pay attention to the care you get. Always make sure you're getting the right treatments and medicines by the right health-care professionals. Don't assume anything."

When to speak-up? There is no definitive test, but there are some key junctures when a patient or advocate always should raise questions. Whenever a medicine is going to be administered, ask *Why? What is it? What's the dosage?*

Similarly, when removed from the room for a test or procedure, ask why, what it is, and what the expected benefit is. When transferring floors, say to or from the ICU, ask why, and get assurance that no tube, line, or catheter is left in. Never allow anything to happen such as taking a medication, going for a test, having a procedure, or inserting a line without the patient being named out loud. If for some reason the nurse, doctor, phlebotomist (blood drawer), or other staff person does not state the patient's name, supply it and insist that the provider swipe the patient's wristband and announce the name. Out loud.

Teach back: Finally, patients may be in the position with or without advocates or care givers to administer their own treatment, meaning medications, wound care, injections, physical therapy, or diet. This is a pivotal moment that often begins at discharge and continues in the community, in rehabilitation, or in a nursing home.

Most famous for his guidance "On Telling the Truth" except in limited areas where the practitioners discern that patients do not wish to hear certain bad news, the late internist and ethicist Mack Lipkin, who studied doctor/patient communications, reported that: "the average American physician conducts between 140–160,000 medical interviews in a practice lifetime, making it the most frequently used medical procedure." Medical communications historically have been handled so poorly that about 40 to 80 percent of the conveyed material is quickly forgotten by patients who incorrectly recall almost half of the information that they hear.

In a 1999 survey of over 3,500 decisions that patients made during clinical discussions with doctors, analysts found that only 9 percent of the choices met the "most basic definition of fully informed." The others lacked information about "the nature of the decision," "a patient role in decision-making," or an "exploration of patient preferences."

Relationship and communications breakdowns not only cause errors but come back to plague practitioners in terms of lawsuits. At a conference at Johns Hopkins on "Patient Centered Care," the participants, mainly nurses, were informed that 26 percent of malpractice cases involved the "dysfunctional delivery of information," and 42 percent resulted from either not understanding or "devaluing" patient and family views.

According to George Bernard Shaw, as the Hopkins participants were told, "the single biggest problems in communications is the illusion that it has taken place." While a failure to communicate in a theater may annoy an audience, the same in medicine can ravage a patient.

Providers unfortunately thwart people who want to give them information. Another *JAMA* study found that during crucial initial appointments patients did not succeed in stating concerns 72 percent of the time before physicians interrupted them, which amazingly happened after an average of twenty-three seconds, even though patients needed only an additional six seconds to deliver the information. Patients and their advocates politely should ask providers not to interrupt and to listen. Given rising sensitivity to this issue in health care, providers probably will comply.

What else can doctors to do to spur the flow of critical content? One technique involves setting the agenda for the meeting; in other words, planning for delivery of information on necessary points. A plan should be reached that prioritizes problems such as which ones require tests today, and which others require follow-up visits.

The patient's own perspectives on what could be the problem as well as whatever he has done to cope with it, how he feels any treatments or medicines are working, and probably above all what are his hopes and goals all need to be explored.

Since many practices, clinics, and HMOs schedule tightly and limit encounters to minutes, it makes sense to dispense with pleasantries, social chit-chat, and idle kibitzing while moving to the meat of the meeting with questions like: "What are your concerns or what is troubling you?" It is equally important to keep asking until the patient unpacks all health problems using simple probes like "anything else?"

Providers still need to be empathic. Maya Angelou's dictum that "I have learned that people will forget what you said, people will forget what you did, but will never forget how you made them feel," now is as much a part of the error-fighting canon as Chesley Sullenberger's maxims on cockpit cooperation. the *Journal of the American Medical Association* reported that visits with "misused empathic opportunities" occur over 70 percent of the time and actually take about three minutes longer than appointments with empathy.

■

It is no secret that patients can contribute to medical errors by missing appointments, over or under medicating themselves, failing to immunize, eating or drinking destructively or otherwise. However, providers should "resist the righting-reflex," the natural urge to correct patients, recount their faults, or—worse—moralizing such as by saying that if they continue to miss appointments they will get sicker and be no good to their families.

Perceived as lecturing or chiding, that kind of speech becomes dysfunctional. It tends to make people more resistant to advice and less honest going forward. Mary Catherine Beach, an internist at Hopkins and expert on medical communications, indicates that it is better for the relationship when providers adopt the patients' perspective. For instance, a doctor could say: "It sounds like your life just got so stressful for a time that you just didn't have time to come to your appointments. It just fell to the bottom of your priority list."

More errors are made when patients feel powerless over their care. So empowering patients through training and education, as well as helping them find a comfort level with their treatment tasks is vital. For in-patients, "yes" answers to all three of the following questions have been associated with favorable clinical outcomes:

1. Are my needs being met in the hospital?
2. Am I involved in my care?
3. Am I prepared to care for my condition at home?

Above all, doctors, nurses, and pharmacists should not simply tell patients what to do. The lower the medical literacy of patients and the higher the complexity of the information, the greater the chance that instructions will be forgotten or mangled.

Communication necessitates comprehension, which in turn requires "assessment" typically with a method called "teach back" where patients are asked repeatedly if necessary to restate the nature of their condition, their course of treatment, and especially how and when they will take their medications. Teach back correlates with better patient outcomes. One of its methods, "Ask me 3," calls for patients to present providers with these questions: "What is my main problem? What do I need to do? Why is it important for me to do this?" After getting the answers, the patients teach them back. Patients and advocates who have the most problems with teach back, especially at discharge, are also giving evidence that they will need the most help with continuing care in the form of follow-up calls and visits from nurses and doctors who do not want these people to lose the benefits of their treatment, be harmed, or bounce-back.

While medical errors have not yet started to shrink as a catastrophic social burden, hospitals, doctors, and nurses can curb most of them. Even diagnostic errors likely will fall when hardy methods like teamwork, checklists, structured communications, less reliance on individual memory and more on systems, openness and oversight, and unfettered electronic records ultimately kick in.

Providers mainly know what to do about errors. Our job is to hold their feet to the fire. Force them to make safety a—no, *the*—priority, and teach back to them medicine's hard won lessons, individually as patients and collectively as prudent but frightened consumers, until we can feel secure in their care.

Glossary of Terms and Acronyms Used in Health Care

ACS — American College of Surgeons.

Acute Care Facility — A hospital.

ADE — Adverse Drug Event. An injury or reactions from medication use.

ACGME — Accreditation Counsel for Graduate Medical Education. A private body that sets nation-wide standards for residences and accredits individual hospital programs.

AHRQ — Agency for Healthcare Research and Quality. A federal agency in the Department of Health and Human Services that tracks trends in the provision of medical care across race, class, and regional lines, and funds safety studies.

ASC — Ambulatory Surgery Center. A setting often outside of a hospital where surgical procedures are performed and the patient leaves that day.

ASRS — Aviation Safety Reporting System. The error and incident reporting commission administered by the Federal Aviation Administration (FAA).

BCMA — Bar Code Medication Administration.

BMJ — *British Medical Journal*. A leading medical journal that publishes significant studies.

Bounce-backs — Readmissions to hospitals within thirty days signifying probable medical errors. Medicare will not pay for some Bounce-backs forcing hospitals to pay these costs.

CABG — Coronary Artery Bypass Graft. A surgical heart procedure to bypass a clogged or closed artery.

CAM — Confusion Assessment Method. The main simple test for patient delirium.

CAUTI — Catheter-Associated Urinary Tract Infection.

CDC — Centers for Disease Control and Prevention. The federal agency in the Department of Health and Human Services that sets standards for dealing with forms of disease and infections and monitors and helps control outbreaks.

C. diff. — *Clostridium Difficile*. A hospital-acquired infection that causes severe diarrhea and related symptoms.

CLABSI — Central Line Associated Bloodstream Infection.

CMS — Centers for Medicare & Medicaid Services. The huge agency in the Department of Health and Human Services that finances and administers these public medical insurance programs.

COP — Conditions of Performance. Rules that hospitals must follow on safety and reporting in order to receive Medicare and Medicaid funding.

CPOE — Computerized Physician Order Entry. Electronic ordering by physicians that enters patient medical records and reduces errors due to legibility and cross-checking functions including for drug incompatibility and allergies.

CUSP — Comprehensive Unit-based Safety Program.

Dashboard — A regularly printed and publicly available roster of patient safety information including such events as falls, infections, and surgical errors.

EMR/EHR — Electronic Medical Record, also known as an Electronic Health Record.

FDA — United States Food and Drug Administration, a federal agency in the Department of Health and Human Services.

Five Rights — Rights that patients have from nursing including to the right medication, right dose, at the right time, by the right route, to the right patient.

HAI — Healthcare-Associated Infection or Healthcare-Acquired Infection. Also Hospital-Acquired Infection.

Handoff — An update from one medical professional to another about a patient before the second takes over care.

HIPAA — The Health Insurance Portability and Accountability Act. Enacted by Congress in 1995, it protects the privacy and security of patient records.

HIT — Healthcare Information Technology.

HOB — Head of Bed Elevation. A method of preventing infection when the patient has a central line inserted.

HODAD, Dr. — Hands of death and destruction, a medical menace.

Iatrogenic — A negative outcome from medical care rather than from disease.

ICU — Intensive Care Unit. NICU is neonatal intensive care unit. PICU is pediatric intensive care unit, etc.

IHI — Institute for Healthcare Improvement. A leading private patient safety agency that pioneered electronic trigger tools.

Incident Reporting — The process by which healthcare personnel or electronic systems report events that led to or could lead to negative outcomes for patients.

Informed Consent — The process of healthcare personnel revealing the risks of a treatment or procedure to a patient before the patient agrees to it and undergoes it.

IOM — Institute of Medicine. A component of the National Academy of Sciences.

JAMA — *Journal of the American Medical Association*. A leading medical journal that publishes significant studies and commentary by physicians.

Joint Commission — The principle private accrediting agency of American hospitals.

Long Term Care Facility — A nursing home.

MAR — Medication Administration Record.

Medical Malpractice — Injury to the patient that occurs when treatment falls below the standard of care that the average, prudent practitioner in the community would apply.

Medication Reconciliation (Med Rec) — The process of checking the patient's medicines periodically to see if they are necessary or conflict with each other.

M&M Conference — Morbidity and Mortality Conference. A presentation by physicians on the cause of a complication.

MRSA — Methicillin-Resistant Staphylococcus Aureas. The most common multiple drug-resistant hospital-acquired infection.

NDI — No Touch Disinfection. Advanced automated fogging or ultraviolet methods for disinfection of hospital rooms.

NEJM — *New England Journal of Medicine.* A leading medical journal that publishes significant studies and commentary by physicians.

Never Events — A term pioneered by the National Quality Forum for things that should and must not occur anytime in health care like wrong-site surgery or operating on the wrong patient.

Nosocomial Disease — Disease that occurs in a hospital or clinic.

NPDB — National Practioners Data Bank. A restricted registry of medical malpractice judgments and settlements maintained by the U.S. Department of Health and Human Services.

Patient Safety Organizations — Authorized by AHRQ, these organizations, some public and some private, collect and analyze data, and publish findings with an eye to health-care improvement.

POA — Present on Admission. Conditions, infections, and/or diseases that the patient has when he enters a hospital. Others that he develops in the hospital are mainly considered iatrogenic or caused by care.

Pressure Ulcer — A bedsore.

QAPI — Quality Assessment and Performance Improvement. A unit in a hospital that tracks medical errors. It is a Medicare Condition of Performance (COP).

Rapid Response Team — Also known as a Rapid Response System. These teams respond to a wide variety of acute (sudden) downturns in a patient's condition not limited to cardiac and respiratory arrests. They also respond without going through the normal hierarchy of nurse to resident to attending physician.

Read Back — A system used in healthcare, aviation, and other dangerous industries. In order to assure that the provider understands the particular information, order, prescription, etc., he reads it back to his superior and to the patient to make sure everyone agrees on the content. The patient also may read back instructions. Also known as teach back.

Root Cause Analysis — An interactive process among providers to identify the contributing factors to an adverse event in a patient's treatment.

Sentinel Event — An occurrence in medicine causing death or serious harm to the patient.

Sepsis — A serious systemic infection of the blood stream sometimes known as bacteremia.

SSI — Surgical Site Infection.

Sterilant — A compound intended to kill all microbes in or on a medical instrument.

STS — Society of Thoracic Surgeons.

TDI — Terminal Disinfection. A hospital's protocol for cleaning a room before the next patient occupies it.

Time Outs — Moments before, during, and/or after treatments when providers stop, take stock, and check and double check to assure that they and everyone on the team has done their tasks accurately and properly.

Triggers — Signals in a patient file, now usually electronic, that indicate that a potential error has occurred.

VAP — Ventilator-Associated Pneumonia.

VistA — Veterans Health Information and Technology Architecture. An open-source electronic medical records system developed by the U.S. Veterans Administration and adaptable by other public and private providers.

WHO — World Health Organization. A unit of the United Nations that establishes medical standards including checklists and helps to implement them in cooperating countries.

Workarounds — Shortcuts that health-care personnel use to avoid full compliance with safe procedures or methods.

Endnotes

INTRODUCTION: FULL DISCLOSURE

To Err Is Human: Building a Safer Health System (National Academy Press, 1999) is the seminal modern work on medical error. It summarizes and reports much of the research until the date of its publication. It is published by the Committee on Quality of Healthcare in America of the Institute of Medicine. It contains a trove of statistics and suggestions for improving patient safety mainly in hospital environments.

CHAPTER 1: MEDIAGENIC CASES

For the Libby Zion case and its impact on graduate medical education I used a host of sources including Robert M. Wachter, M.D., *Understanding Patient Safety* (2nd Edition, Mcgraw-Hill Lange, 2012) and Marty Makary, M.D., *Unaccountable: What Hospitals Won't Tell You and How Transparency Can Revolutionize Health Care* (Bloomsbury, 2012). A great deal of important journalism also emanated from the case including "A Case That Shook Medicine" by Barron H. Lerner, M.D., *The Washington Post* (November 28, 2006); "The Legacy of Libby Zion," *New York Times* (June 8, 1987); "The Obituary of Libby Zion," *New York Times* (March 6, 1984); an obituary by Robert D. McFadden (August 3, 2009): "Sidney Zion, Writer Who Crusaded to Reduce Doctors' Hours Dies at 75;" "A Life Changing Case for Doctors in Training," by Barron H. Lerner M.D., *New York Times* (March 3, 2009). Another extensive piece about Sidney Zion appears in *Tablet: A New Read on Jewish Life: "El Sid"* by Victor Navasky (August 12, 2009). For an obituary of Elsa Zion see "Elsa Zion, 70, Helped Cut Doctor Work Loads," *New York Times* (March 5, 2005). I also reviewed trial testimony and legal material from *Zion v. New York Hospital* at law.jrank. org/pages/3630.

For a more technical approach to improving the condition of residents see "Beyond Duty Hour Reform: Redefining the Learning Environment," in a report of *The Association of Program Directors in Internal Medicine* (APDIM) by Lisa M. Bellini, M.D., et al. (March 2009). Also see Gregory S. Cherr, M.D., "The Origins of Regulated Resident Work Hours: New York and Beyond," *Bulletin of The American College of Surgeons* (November 2002).

For the material that appears on Betsy Lehman and Dana-Farber Cancer Center, I utilized Susan Brink "Tragedy at Dana-Farber: Betsy Lehman's Shocking Death is Still Roiling the Medical Community," *US News and World Report* (July 16, 1995); "Hospital Rocked by Health Columnist's Death," *Reading Eagle/Reading Times Associated Press* (March 24, 1994). The same source reported "Girl Dies After Routine Tonsillectomy." Also see Scott Allen "With Work, Dana-Farber Learns From '94 Mistakes," *Boston Globe* (November 30, 2004); Lawrence K. Altman "Big Doses of Chemotherapy Drug Killed Patient, Hurt Second," *New York Times* (March 24, 1995). Another Institute of Medicine publication *Preventing Medication Errors* published by the National Academies Press analyzed the Lehman case at box 1 on page 27.

Also see "A Cancer Patient Killed By Carelessness," *Boston Globe* (March 30, 1995); Lucian L. Leape "A Blueprint on Patient Safety," *Boston.com* (November 15, 2011). I also perused the Betsy Lehman Center for Patient Safety and Medical Error Reduction, a service of the Commonwealth of Massachusetts http://chiamass.gov/betsy-lehman-center. Another useful analysis appeared in *Web M&M: Morbidity and Mortality Rounds on the Web* produced by the Agency for Healthcare Research and Quality (AHRQ) of the United States Department of Health and Human Services. A key article is Conway and Weingart, "Organizational Change in the Face of Highly Public Errors I. The Dana-Farber Cancer Institute Experience."

For the Willie King case I made use of Mike Clary, "Strings of Errors Put Florida Hospital on The Critical List" *Los Angeles Times* (April 14, 1995); "Hospital Settles Case of Amputation Error," *New York Times* (May 12, 1995); "Doctor Who Cut Off Wrong Leg is Defended by Colleagues," *New York Times* (September 17, 1995).

For an excellent article on how the Willie King case and other cases like it created reforms to prevent wrong-site surgery, see "Reducing the Risk of Wrong-Site Surgery" by the Joint Commission Center for Transforming Healthcare (May 13, 2013).

For the Jesica Santillan tragedy and the cases related to it, I drew upon the following articles, David Resnick "The Jesica Santillan Tragedy: Lessons Learned" *The Hastings Center Report* (July through August 2003) pages 15–20; Lawrence K. Altman "Even the Elite Hospitals Aren't Immune to Errors," *New York Times* (February 23, 2003); "Teen's Family Grateful After 2nd Transplant," *CNN.com* (February 21, 2003); Ellen Goodman "Doctors Must Battle 'Banality of Screw-Up'," *Boston Globe* (February 28, 2003). Randall C. Archibold "Girl in Transplant Mix-up Dies After Two Weeks," *New York Times* (February 23, 2003); Laura Mechler "Girls Death Spurs New Transplant Rules," *Associated Press* (June 29, 2003); Denise Grady and Lawrence K. Altman "Suit Says Transplant Error Was Cause In Baby's Death," *New York Times* (March 12, 2003); and Sheryl Gay Stolberg "Transplant Mix-Up Enters Debate in Congress on Malpractice Bills," *New York Times* (February 26, 2003). In addition, I obtained James Jaggers M.D., "Lessons Learned From a 'Botched' Transplant," *Presentation to the Third Annual Betsy Lehman Center Patient Safety Conference*. The Santillan case also was addressed in Robert M. Wachter "Understanding Patient Safety," McGraw-Hill Lange 2nd Edition, page 5.

CHAPTER 2: HOPKINS, HISTORY, AND MEDICAL ERRORS
There were many excellent articles on the Josie King tragedy. Sorrell King's story "Life After Josie" (*Good Housekeeping, October 2009*) links the themes of what went wrong to what a family can do about the safety of its child. The *Baltimore Sun* carried an extensive two-part series on the case. See Erika Niedowski "A Mother's Promise: How Medical Errors Took a Little Girl's Life," *Baltimore Sun* (December 14, 2003); and Erika Niedowski "A Mother's Promise: From Tragedy, A Quest for Safer Care," *Baltimore Sun* (December 15, 2003). Johns Hopkins also published its own analysis. See Mary Ann Ayd "A Remedy of Errors," *Hopkins Medicine* (Spring/Summer 2004). The introduction to *Safe Patients, Smart Hospitals* by Peter Pronovost M.D., PhD and Eric Vohr, Plume 1973 specifically deals with the Josie King case and how it transformed medical safety at Johns Hopkins and elsewhere. *Josie's Story: A Mother's Inspiring Crusade to Make Medical Care Safe* by Sorrel

King, Grove Press New York (2009), is among the best and most moving memoirs of medical errors. Further it details many reforms that have been implemented to make hospitals safer as well as Sorrel King's dedication to both stopping and revealing medical errors at Hopkins.

For histories of the great medical pioneers at Johns Hopkins I drew upon *The Cambridge Illustrated History of Medicine*, edited by Roy Porter, Cambridge University Press, 1998 and *The Greatest Benefit to Mankind: A Medical History of Humanity*, by Roy Porter, W.W. Norton (1997). Dr. Pronovost's book also was helpful in terms of understanding medical morality and high level of care at Hopkins. Other useful histories included Erwin H. Ackerknecht M.D., *A Short History of Medicine*, The Johns Hopkins University Press, Revised Edition (1982) and *The History of Medicine, A Very Short Introduction* by William Bynum, Oxford University Press (2008). I also drew upon Mary-Jane Schneider *Introduction to Public Health*, 3rd Edition, Jones and Bartlett Publishers LLC. (2011), which is an excellent introduction to historical community health strides as well as to the larger social context of medical advances.

CHAPTER 3: BAD DOCTORS, NEWSMAKERS, AND CELEBRITIES

An excellent report on bad doctors as well as the portion of mistakes that they cause is "Medical Negligence: The Role of America's Civil Justice System in Protecting Patients' Rights," *American Association for Justice* (February 2011). Some of these cases also generated news articles upon which I drew. For Andy Warhol, these included "Treatment of Warhol is Defended" by Steven Lee Myers, *New York Times* (December 6, 1991) and "Care Faulted In the Death of Warhol" by Ronald Sullivan, *New York Times* (December 5, 1991).

For the Dana Carvey case see "The Heart of The Matter" by Susan Schindehette, *People* (June 5, 2000). On the situation involving the Quaid twins see "Why Dennis Quaid is Fighting To Improve Patient Safety" by Tiffany O'Callaghan, *Time* (April 23, 2010). Also see "Preventable Medical Malpractice: Revisiting the Dennis Quaid Medication/Hospital Error Case" by Rick Shapiro, *The Legal Examiner* (Virginia) (August 9, 2010). For the treatment of the Shah of Iran see "The Shah's Spleen: Its Impact on History" by Leon Morganstern, M.D., FACS, in the *Journal of the American College of Surgeons* (September 2, 2010). Also see "The Shah's Health: A Political Gamble" by Lawrence K. Altman, M.D., *The New York Times* (May

17, 1981). For the Michael Skolnik case see "A Profile of Patty Skolnik," his mother, the Founder and Executive Director of Citizens for Patient's Safety produced by the Consumer's Union. Also see "Family's Fight for Malpractice Disclosure Keeps Son's Memory Alive" by Peter Jones, *Colorado Community Newspapers* (June 7, 2007). The Skolnik Law is found at Colorado Revised Statutes Title 24 Professions and Occupations Article 34 Department of Regulatory Agencies Effective July 1, 2011 (24-34-110). Formally known as the Medical Transparency Act of 2010—Disclosure of Information About Healthcare Licensees—Fines—Rules—Short Title—Legislative Declaration effective July 1, 2011. Also see "10 Doctors Who Shamed Their Profession" in http://www.mastersinhealthcare.com/blog/2011/10-doctors-who-shamed-their-profession/.

In *Unaccountable: What Hospitals Won't Tell You and How Transparency Can Revolutionize Healthcare* by Marty Makary M.D., Bloomsbury Press, 2012, bad doctoring is described from this leading surgeon's perspective in a variety of cases including those of Carvey, Skolnik, and Warhol. Dr. Makary deserves credit for injecting the term "Dr. HODAD" meaning "hands of death and destruction" into the public dialogue on the errors question. Dr. Makary also analyses the care of the Shah of Iran and the deficient surgical performance of Dr. Michael DeBakey, the leading surgeon of the era. Makary discusses some principles that are now becoming better recognized including the level of experience in particular procedures including his own (pancreatic surgery). Other good books bearing on bad doctors include: William Charney, *Epidemic of Medical Errors and Hospital Acquired Infections: Systemic and Social Causes*. CRC Press (2012); Otis Webb Brawley, M.D., with Paul Goldberg, *How We Do Harm: A Doctor Breaks Ranks About Being Sick In America*, St. Martin's Press (2011); and Shannon Brownlee, *Overtreated: Why Too Much Medicine is Making Us Sicker and Poorer*, Bloomsbury (2008).

CHAPTER 4: OUR ATTITUDES CHANGE

For this chapter I found Peter Pronovost's book *Safe Patients, Smart Hospitals* helpful. In addition, the 1999 Institute of Medicine (IOM) Report *To Err Is Human: Building a Safer Health System* likewise pointed me to issues on rising levels of error in healthcare. In addition there are important survey articles. See "Five Years After IOM Report on Medical Errors, Nearly Half of All Consumers Worry About the Safety of Their Healthcare," by the Henry J. Kaiser Family Foundation (November 15, 2004). The Kaiser Family Foundation, The Agency for Healthcare Research and Quality in the Harvard Medical School and School of Public Health put together the important "National Survey on Consumers' Experiences with Patient Safety and Quality Information," (November 20, 2004). Also see "Survey Shows Fear of Medical Errors" by Ceci Connolly, *Washington Post* (November 18, 2004). For an extensive analysis pointing to a variety of polls see "Americans' Views of Healthcare Costs, Access and Quality" by Robert J. Blendon, et al. in *The Milbank Quarterly*, Vol. 84, no. 4 (2006). Also see "Healthcare and Public Opinion" by Michael J. Pentecost, M.D., in *The Permanente Journal* (Summer 2006), Vol. 10, no. 2. For a survey of rising concerns of parents regarding the hospitalizations of their children see a study by Beth A. Tarini, M.D., M.S. in the July 30, 2009 *Journal of Hospital Medicine* that pertained to the Children's Hospital and Regional Medical Center in Seattle Washington. Also see "A Community Survey of Medical Errors in New York" by Richard E. Adams and Joseph A. Boscarino in the *International Journal for Quality in Health Care*, Vol. 16 no. 5 (2004); "Report on Americans' Views on The Quality of Healthcare" by R. J. Blendon, et al. for the Harvard School of Public Health (March 2011). For a survey on patient concerns about being harmed in hospitals see "Consumer Reports Poll Finds High Levels of Concern About Medical Harm and Support for Public Ratings on Hospital Safety" (March 31, 2011). For perceptions of Americans on healthcare see "The Robert Wood Johnson Foundation Healthcare Public Perception Index," (April 2011) report. For how Americans perceive healthcare quality, particularly individuals with household incomes less than $50,000, see "When it Comes to Quality, New Poll Shows Americans Give U.S. Healthcare Low Grades," *Harvard School of Public Health News* (April 12, 2011). Regarding satisfaction or lack thereof with the healthcare system see "Americans Maintain Negative View of U.S. Healthcare Coverage," *Gallup Health and Healthcare Survey* (November 16, 2011) by Lydia Saad. Also see "Medical Errors Continue to Dog Healthcare" by Madelyn Kerns in *Healthcare IT News* (August 17, 2012) describing a Wolters-Kluwer survey of a thousand U.S. consumers. For attitudes on technology in healthcare see "Patients Believe Tech Can Fix Medical Errors, Says Survey" (August 20, 2012) in Healthcare-Informatics.com (August 20, 2012). Patient experiences were reported in "Medical Mistakes Affect One in Three Individuals," by Emily Mullen in PatientAdvocateTraining.com (August 22, 2012). The degree of apprehension about medical errors was summed in *American Medical News* of the American Medical Association in an article by Kevin B. O'Reilly, "Seventy-Three Percent of Patients Worry About Medical Errors, Poll Says" (September 4, 2012). Regarding the fears of women giving birth see "National Survey Finds Moms Face Many Physical and Emotional Challenges After Birth; Many Have Concerns About Injury From Medical Errors While in the Hospital for Birth," Reuters.com (June 11, 2013). The article reported a survey of over one thousand polled about post-partum experiences and views of maternity care.

CHAPTER 5: SIZING THE PROBLEM

The number of medical errors and deaths in the U.S. health-care system has spawned a great deal of reporting. In particular I was informed by "How Many Die From Medical Mistakes in U.S. Hospitals" by Marshall Allen, *ProPublica* (September 19, 2013) and "Temporal Trends and Rates of Patient Harm Resulting From Patient Care," by C. P. Landrigan, et al., *New England Journal of Medicine* (November 24, 2010). Regarding global trigger measurement techniques see "Global Trigger Tool Shows That Adverse Events in Hospitals May Be Ten Times Greater Than Previously Measured," by David C. Classen, et al. in *Health Affairs* (April 2011), and "IHI Global Trigger Tool for Measuring Adverse Events" by the Institute for Healthcare Improvement (undated, last modified August 13, 2013); David Classen, et al. "Development and Evaluation of The Institute For Healthcare Improvement Global Trigger Tool," in *The Journal of Patient Safety* (September 4, 2008). The size of the modern problem first was analyzed in *To Err is Human: Building a Safer Health System*, by the Institute of Medicine (1999). Basic to this study was "The Nature of Adverse Events in Hospitalized Patients," by Lucian L. Leape, M.D., et al., *New England Journal of Medicine*, Vol. 324, no. 6 (February 7, 1991). Likewise see "Identification of Adverse Events Occurring During Hospitalization: A Cross-Sectional Study of Litigation, Quality, Assurance and Medical Records at Two Teaching Hospitals," by Troyen A. Brennan M.D., et al., in the *Annals of Internal Medicine* (February 1, 1990). The study on which the previous article was based is Troyen A. Brennan M.P.H. M.D., J.D., et al. "Incidents of Adverse Events and Negligence in Hospitalized Patients, Results of the Harvard Medical Practice Study No. 1," *New England Journal of Medicine* (February 7, 1991). Another study from HealthGrades was reported in "In Hospital Deaths From Medical Errors at 195,000 Per Year," in *Medical News Today* (August 9, 2004). Regarding juvenile deaths see "Small Patients, Big Consequences in Medical Errors," in *The New York Times* (September 15, 2008). Regarding Medicare patients and the numbers hurt during hospitalization and the Office of Inspector General of Health and Human Services study see "Mistakes Chronicled on Medicare Patients," by Duff Wilson, *The New York Times* (November 15, 2010). For a conversation between two pioneering patient-safety experts on the nature and the scope of the problem I obtained a transcript from the PBS Newshour "Dr. Wachter and Dr. Leape On Medical Errors" that aired on February 7, 2005; Robert Wachter and Lucian Leape discussed progress since the publication of the IOM Report. Dr. Leape was interviewed by Tony A. Augillo in a Clinical Resources Podcast January 1, 2010. For deaths by other causes I also viewed The Centers for Disease Control and Prevention "Leading Causes of Death," from 2010 forward.

Regarding misdiagnosis see "Misdiagnosis is More Common Than Drug Errors or Wrong-Site Surgery," by Sandra G. Boodman, *The Washington Post* (May 6, 2013), " 'Misdiagnosis' Leading Cause of U.S. Malpractice Payouts: Study," by Denise Mann in *U.S. News and World Report* (April 22, 2013). Also see "Diagnostic Errors Are the Most Common Type of Medical Mistake," by Alexandra Sifferlin, *Time* (April 24, 2013) and "Diagnostic Errors more Common, Costly and Harmful Than Treatment Mistakes," *(e) Science News* (April 23, 2013). I spoke with Dr. Peter Pronovost on the total size and types of medical errors on August 23, 2013. I heard him speak on this and other topics including patient safety at Johns Hopkins on September 23, 2013. For a good piece on autopsies as an estimating tool see "Diagnostic Errors in The Intensive Care Unit: A Systematic Review of Autopsy Studies," by Bradford Winters et al., *BMJ Quality and Safety* Online (July 21, 2012).

CHAPTER 6: MACRO AND MICRO

Diagnostic error is an emerging field of research. In particular, I was informed by "Diagnostic Error in Medicine: Analysis of 583 Physician-Reported Errors," by Gordon D. Schiff M.D., et al., in the *Archives of Internal Medicine*, Vol. 169 No. 20 (November 9, 2009), "Why Diagnostic Errors Don't Get Any Respect . . . And What Can Be Done About It," By Robert

Wachter in the-hospitalist.org (June 2, 2008), "Physician Perspectives on Preventing Diagnostic Errors," by Owen J. McDonald in *QuantiaMD*, "Diagnostic Error in Medicine: Introduction," by Eta S. Berner in Springer Science+Business Media B.V. (August 11, 2009), "Diagnostic Error: Is Overconfidence the Problem?" edited by Mark L. Graber, M.D., and Eta S. Berner in *The American Journal of Medicine* (May 2008) Vol. 121.

Probably the most significant study of diagnostic errors published in this century is "25-year Summary of Malpractice Claims for Diagnostic Errors 1986–2010: An Analysis from the National Practitioner Data Bank," by A. S. Saber Tehrani, HeeWon Lee, Simon C. Matthews, Andrew Shore, Martin Makary, Peter J. Pronovost, and David E. Newman-Toker, all of Johns Hopkins. This article appeared in *BMJ (British Medical Journal) Quality and Safety* (April 22, 2013). Another important study based at Hopkins is "Diagnostic Errors in the Intensive Care Unit: A Systematic Review of Autopsy Studies," by Bradford Winters, et al. that appeared in *BMJ Quality and Safety* (July 21, 2012). A particularly prescient article on the misdiagnosis/medical error problem is "Diagnostic Errors—The Next Frontier For Patient Safety," by David E. Newman-Toker, M.D., Ph.D. and Peter J. Provonost, M.D., Ph.D. in the *Journal of the American Medical Association* (March 10, 2009).

I interviewed Dr. Newman-Toker about diagnostic errors and stroke detection on December 2, 2013 at the Bloomberg School of Public Health, I was further informed by other articles which he wrote or to which he contributed including "How Much Diagnostic Safety Can We Afford, And How Should We Decide? A Health Economics Perspective," in *BMJ Quality and Safety* (August 8, 2013) and "Measuring Diagnostic Errors in Primary Care: The First Step On a Path Forward" by Drs. Newman-Toker and Makary in *JAMA Internal Medicine* (March 25, 2013). Also see "Reducing Cognitive Skill Decay and Diagnostic Error: Theory-Based Practices For Continuing Education in Health Care" by Sallie J. Weaver, Ph.D, David E. Newman-Toker, M.D., Ph.D. and Michael A. Rosen, Ph.D. In *The Journal of Continuing Education in the Health Professions* (December 19, 2012), "Diagnostic Errors and Patient Safety," by Robert M. Wachter, M.D., and Eric S. Holmboe, M.D., *Journal of The American Medical Association* (July 15, 2009) and "Cognitive and System Factors Contributing to Diagnostic Errors in Radiology," by Cindy S. Lee, Paul G. Nagy, Sallie J. Weaver, and David E. Newman-Toker in *The American Journal of Roentgenology* (2013 Vol. 201).

On stroke detection I was informed by "Quantitative Video-Oculography to Help Diagnose Stroke in Acute Vertigo and Dizziness, Toward an ECG for the Eyes," by David E. Newman-Toker in *Stroke* (2013); 44: 1158–1161.

CHAPTER 7: THE THIRD LEADING CAUSE OF DEATH

My views in this area were affected by the fine manual by Robert M. Wachter, *Understanding Patient Safety*, McGraw-Hill Lange, 2nd Ed. (2012), by my interviews with Drs. Pronovost and Newman-Toker, and by "A New, Evidence-Based Estimate of Patient Harms Associated With Hospital Care" by John T. James, Ph.D. in *The Journal of Patient Safety*, Vol. 9 No. 3 (September 2013). Also see a conversation with David C. Classen, M.D., M.S. in *Agency for Healthcare Research and Quality: Morbidity and Mortality.* AHRQ WebM&M Podcast May 2012. Classen is probably the leading developer of global trigger tools to estimate medical errors.

For adverse drug events as a form of errors see "Adverse Drug Events in Hospitalized Patients: Excess Length of Stay, Extra Costs and Attributable Mortality," by Classen, et al. in the *Journal of The American Medical Association* (January 22, 1997). For a lawyer's perspective see "Medical Errors Continue to Be Problematic" in *Lexology* (August 1, 2013). *The U.S. News and World Report* Health Online Edition covered the issue in "Medical Errors Harm Huge Number of Patients," by Steve Sternberg (August 28, 2012). *ProPublica* reported on it in "How Many Die From Medical Mistakes in U.S. Hospitals?" by Marshall Allen. William Charney M.D., makes the case for medical errors being probably the leading cause of death in the United States. See the book *Epidemic of Medical Errors in Hospital-Acquired Infections: Systemic and Social Causes*, edited by William Charney and see his article "Do No Harm" (July 2012) in *Z Magazine* where he estimates 788,000 deaths per year. In *Patient Safety Focus*, a blog, this number was estimated at an average of 195,000 people dying of preventable in-hospital medical errors as was found by *HealthGrades*. For a strong contrarian view in the wake of the IOM study see "Deaths Due to Medical Errors Are Exaggerated in Institute of Medicine Report" by Clement J. McDonald, M.D., in the *Journal of The American Medical Association* (July 5, 2000). For a good piece on how misdiagnosis affects these numbers see "Johns Hopkins Team Finds ICU Misdiagnosis May Account For As Many Annual Deaths As Breast Cancer," a press release by the Armstrong Institute (August 27, 2012). The Pronovost-led efforts to reduce central line infections were detailed in his book *Safe Patients, Smart Hospitals.* He also detailed these results in a September 2013 Patient Safety Conference at Johns Hopkins and compared medical error to other leading causes of death. Martin Makary M.D., made a case for medical errors and preventable infections being the third leading cause of death in the United States to the Sub-committee on Energy Policy, Health Care and Entitlements of the Committee on Oversight and Government Reform of the House of Representatives on August 25, 2013 in a session entitled "Examining the Lack of Transparency and Consumer-Driven Market Forces in US Healthcare" available at *oversight. house.gov.* William Charney M.D., laid out his case for why medical error is the first leading cause of death in *Z Magazine* on September 12, 2012 in an article entitled "The Carnage Continues, Part II." A good article on medical error in another advanced society is "The Incidence and Nature of In-Hospital Adverse Events: A Systemic Review" by E. N. de Vries that appeared in *Quality Safety Health Care* 2008; 17: 216–223. The article dealt with eight studies in the Netherlands covering over 70,000 patients and finding an adverse event rate in hospitals of 9.2% with a median preventability rate of 43.5%. For more on relevant causes of death see Ian R. H. Rockett, Ph.D., M.P.H., et al., "Leading Causes of Unintentional and Intentional Injury Mortality: United States, 2000–2009" in *The American Journal of Public Health* (November 2012), Vol. 102, no. 11 and see the graphic "Ten Leading Causes of Injury Deaths By Age Group Highlighting Unintentional Injury Deaths, United States–2010" by *The Centers for Disease Control and Prevention,* National Center for Injury Prevention and Control. For more on staffing ratios, a problem that Charney has focused on, see Paul G. Shekelle, M.D., PhD "Nurse–Patient Ratios As A Patient Safety Strategy: A Systematic Review" Annals of Internal Medicine (March 5, 2013) Vol. 158 No. 5. Regarding the problems suffered by Medicare patients the best report is "Adverse Events in Hospitals: National Incidence Among Medicare Beneficiaries," by Daniel R Levinson, Inspector General, Department of Health and Human Services (November 2010).

CHAPTER 8: THE NEEDLESS PREVALENCE OF MEDICATION ERRORS
For this chapter, I was informed about the Vasquez case, look-alike and sound-alike drugs, medical administration, dosing, and some aspects of clinical pharmacy by Robert M. Wachter's *Understanding Patient Safety, 2nd Edition* McGraw-Hill (2012). These topics also are covered in depth in

a publication of The Institute of Medicine: *Preventing Medication Errors*, edited by Phillip Espden et al. (2007). Charting and medication errors including from look-alike drugs appear in *Mastering Medical Records* by Samuel D. Hodge, Jr., of Temple University, published by The Pennsylvania Bar Institute in 2014, also see the "Do Not Use List of Abbreviations," published by the Joint Commission in 2001. For a report on declines in errors following the implementation of preventive strategies see "Dramatic Reductions in Medication Errors Reported at International Patient Safety Conference," and EurekALERT! by *The American Association for the Advancement of Science* (November 9, 1998), "Preventing Medical Errors: A $21 Billion Opportunity," by *The National Priorities Partnership/National Quality Forum* (December 2010) and in Mayo Clinic Consumer Health (October 15, 2011). *The Annals of Internal Medicine* published a supplement on the topic, "Medication Reconciliation During Transitions of Care as a Patient Safety Strategy: A Systematic Review," by Janice L. Kwan, M.D., et al., Annals of Internal Medicine 2013; 158: 397–403. For the major study of the efficacy of clinical pharmacy see "Medication Errors in United States Hospitals," by C. A. Bond, et al. in *Pharmacotherapy*, 2001; 21(9). An important article on misprescribing in a hospital setting is "Adverse Drug Events in Hospitalized Patients: Excess Length of Stay, Extra Costs, and Attributable Morality," by David C. Classen, M.D., et al., in the *Journal of The American Medical Association* (January 22–29 1997). The Food & Drug Administration has various regulations to prevent misleading labeling: 21 CFR 201.1 (C) and 21 CFR 201.6 (B) and also has developed guidance on naming, labeling, and packaging to reduce errors. See /drugs/NewsEvents/ ucm214703.htm. Regarding care transitions "Medication Discrepancies in Residents Sign-Outs and Their Potential to Harm," by Vineet Arora, M.D., MA et al. in *The Journal of Geriatric Internal Medicine* (October 26, 2007). A good piece on nurses using electronic strategies such as bar coding is "Implementation of an Electronic Medication Administration Record and Bedside Verification System," by Karen M. Hunter, R.N., B.S.N. in the online Journal of Nursing Informatics (July 2, 2011) (OJNI), 15(2), available at *http:// ojni.org/issues/?p=672*. Also see "Medication Errors: Don't Let Them Happen To You," by Pamela Anderson, M.S., R.N, CCRN and Terri Townsend, M.A., R.N., CCRN in *American Nurse Today* (March 2010).

For reasons why errors still occur with bar-coding see "Medication Errors Occurring With The Use of Bar-Code Administration Technology," in *Pennsylvania Patient Safety Advisory* (December 5, 2008). The same publication, an official outlet of the State of Pennsylvania, produced "Wrong-Patient Medication Errors Examined by the Pennsylvania Patient Safety Authority," (June 3, 2013). For background on the evolution of the corporation Barcoding Inc., a US Patent holder which also produces radio frequency identification devices (RFID) see "A CEO Conversation With Jay Steinmetz, CEO and Founder of Barcoding, Inc.," by Offit Kurman Attorneys at Law (*www.offitkurman.com*), April 22, 2014 published online. For a brief history of checking in the banking industry see "The History of the Checking Account," by Erin O'Neil in *www.banks.com* (August 1, 2012).

CHAPTER 9: THE DREAM AND TRAGEDY OF ELECTRONIC MEDICAL ERRORS
This is a huge topic, the amount of coverage is large and much of it is basically in the vein of public relations and should be read skeptically. However, there were a number of articles in journals, news outlets, and government sources that I found useful to writing this chapter and I will try to at least present some of them.

A very interesting article is "Barriers for Adopting Electronic Health Records (EHRs) By Physicians," by Sema Ajami and Tayyede Bagheri-Tadi in *Acta Inform Medicine* (June 2013). These individuals are at Isfahan University of Medical Sciences in Iran, and they describe benefits and advantages of electronic medical records that transcend cultural barriers. Also see "A Digital Shift on Health Data Swell Profits in an Industry," by Julie Creswell, *New York Times* (February 19, 2013), "Using Electronic Health Records to Improve Quality and Efficiency: The Experiences of Leading Hospitals," by Sharon Silow-Carroll et al., *The Commonwealth Fund* (July 2012), "Identifying Diagnostic Errors in Primary Care Using Electronic Screening Algorithm," by Hardeep Singh M.D., M.P.H. et al. in the *Journal of The American Medical Association* (February 12, 2007). Dr. Singh is one of the most trenchant thinkers on electronic medical records and trigger tools.

See "Mining Electronic Records For Revealing Health Data," by Peter Jaret, *New York Times* (January 14, 2013) and "The Benefits of Mobile Health, On Hold," by Tina Rosenberg, *New York Times* (March 13, 2013). This is a good piece on the important potential interface between electronic medical records and cell phones that is especially promising in underdeveloped environments.

Also see "The Value From Investments In Health Information Technology At The US Department of Veterans Affairs," published in *Health Affairs* (April 2010). This is an official release by the VA and introduces its computerized patient record system, its barcode medication administration (BCMA), and the VistA system. For a good short piece on how the introduction of medical records wreaked havoc on family practitioners see "The EHR Incentive Program: Consider Waiting For Next Year" by David C. Kibbe M.D., in *FamilyDoctor.Org* (July 7, 2011). For fine coverage of the rise of the VA and its electronic record system VistA see "The Best Care Anywhere," by Phillip Longman in *The Washington Monthly* (January/February 2005). For reporting on the American electronic medical records market see "US Market for Electronic Medical Records," *PRN Newswire* (November 28, 2012) and "EHR Market To Reach 6.5 Billion By 2012," by Nicole Lewis in *Information Week* (October 21, 2011). For a piece on the expense of dealing with medical records giants see "Considering an Epic Journey in 2013? Think Twice," posted by Edmund Billings M.D., on December 6, 2012 in the blog *Medsphere*. For the federal government approach to the problem including by the Obama Administration, Congress, and the industry lobbies see HIMSS, "Health IT Policy and the 111th Congress: 2009 Year in Review" (January 24, 2010). A good blog covering the VistA and world VistA struggle is "Open Source Electronic Health Record Alliance (OSEHRA)," in particular see "Will VistA Be Dashed on the Rocks?" by Nancy Anthracite (October 23, 2012). Also see the WorldVistA website *www.worldvista.org*. For a survey of practitioners using electronic records see "The 2012 EHR User Satisfaction Survey: Responses From 3088 Family Physicians," by Robert L. Edsall and Kenneth G. Adler M.D., in *Family Practice Management* (November–December, 2012).

Regarding the so-called HI TECH Act, which was enacted as part of the American Recovery and Reinvestment Act see "Q4 2012 included Key Federal Health IT Developments," by Helen R. Pfister et al. in *ihealthbeat.org* (January 22, 2013). Recipient data including for the Hi Tech Act can be found at *www.recovery.gov/transparency/recoverydata*. A Rand Corporation Report on Health IT is found in "What Will It Take To Achieve The As-Yet-Unfulfilled Promises Of Health Information Technology," by Arthur J. Kellermann and Spencer S. Jones published in *Health Affairs* (January 2013) Vol. 32 No. 1. For a survey on the evolution of medical records in medicine and the expenses involved see "Effect of Electronic Health

Records on Health Care Costs: Longitudinal Comparative Evidence From Community Practices," by Julia Adler-Milstein, PhD, in *Harvard Medical School Health Care Policy* (July 16, 2013). For a piece that seems to show that electronic medical records are having a good if small effect on patient experiences in hospitals including length of stay and mortality see "The Effect of Electronic Medical Record Adoption on Outcomes in US Hospitals," by Jinhyung Lee et al. in *BMC Health Services Research* (2013) 13:39. Electronic medical records combined with computerized physician order entry (CPOE) also had measurable positive effect in neo-natal care. See "The Electronic Medical Record: Pros and Cons," by Maria Louisa Ventura et al. in *The Journal of Maternal-Fetal and Neonatal Medicine* (2011); 24 (s) 11:163–166. This piece surveys the use of EMR in an Italian maternity hospital. An article concluding that EMR cannot simply be imposed on a hospital but must be customized is "Towards Plug-and-Play Integration of Archetypes Into Legacy Electronic Health Record System: The ArchiMed Experience," by Georg Duftschmid et al. in *BMC Medical Informatics and Decision Making* (2013), 13:11. A United Kingdom study is "The Provision and Impact of Online Patient Access to Their Electronic Health Records (EHR) and Transactional Services on the Quality and Safety of Health Care: Systematic Review Protocol," by Freda Mold et al. in *Informatics In Primary Care* (2012); 20:271–82. I interviewed Carol Zisowitz M.D., PhD, the psychiatrist and critic of the way in which Washington has fostered the adoption of medical records, at various times during December 2014. For an understanding of railroad standardization, see "The Standardization of Track Gauge on North American Railways, 1830–1890," by Douglas J. Puffert in *The Journal of Economic History* Vol. 60 No. 4 (December 2000) pages 933–960.

CHAPTER 10: CENTURIES OF HOSPITAL INFECTIONS

Infectious disease is a massive topic. So again I will list only important sources that helped me to begin to grasp it. For the history of addressing infection including this story of Ignaz Semmelweis I utilized some histories of medicine including *A Short History of Medicine, Revised Edition*, by Erwin H. Ackerknecht, M.D., The Johns Hopkins University Press (1982), *The Greatest Benefit to Mankind: A Medical History of Humanity* by Roy Porter, W.W. Norton & Company (1997) New York and London, and *The Cambridge Illustrated History of Medicine*, edited by Roy Porter, Cambridge

University Press, Cambridge and New York (1998). For society's approach to dealing with infection on a preventative and policy basis I used *Introduction to Public Health*, 3rd Edition, by Mary-Jane Schneider, Jones and Bartlett, Sudbury Massachusetts (2011). I also used some basic medical texts that have guided doctors, medical students, and other health-care professionals. These include *Practical Guide to the Care of the Medical Patient, 3rd Edition* by Fred F. Ferri, Mosby, St. Louis Missouri (1995), *The Washington Manual of Medical Therapeutics, 31st Edition*, by The Department of Medicine, Washington University School of Medicine, St. Louis, Missouri (2004), *The Critical Care Handbook of The Massachusetts General Hospital, 3rd Edition*, published by Lippincott Williams and Wilkens, Philadelphia, Pennsylvania (2000), senior editor William E. Hurford, *Harrison's Manual of Medicine 15th Edition*, McGraw-Hill (2002) and *Cecil Textbook of Medicine, 20th Edition* (1996) edited by J. Claude Bennett, W. B. Saunders Company, Philadelphia, Pennsylvania. I also found *The Medical Knowledge Self-Assessment Program* Vol. 14 on Infectious Disease by The American College of Physicians, Philadelphia (2006) to be especially clear and valuable. One can look up most known infections in this book and learn practical and safe ways for practitioners to deal with it. Much the same can be said for *Understanding Patient Safety 2nd Edition* by Robert M. Wachter M.D., McGraw-Hill Lang (2012) although this manual does not focus specifically on infection but on the myriad problems that patients can experience mainly in the hospital, *The Mayo Clinic Internal Medicine Review 8th Edition*, editor in chief Amit K. Ghosh M.D. (2008) Mayo Clinic Scientific Press, Rochester, Minnesota, is an extremely valuable training tool on all forms of disease including infectious diseases. Peter Pronovost's memoir *Safe Patients, Smart Hospitals, How One Doctor's Checklist Can Help Us Change Health Care from the Inside Out*, clearly recounts the efforts of a critical care (ICU) doctor to simplify and spread his knowledge to the wider fight against man-made infections from in-dwelling catheters, central lines, and ventilators. Regarding hand hygiene and surveillance see "Promotion of Hand Hygiene Technique," *The Journal of Hospital Infection* (June 2007), "Latest Research and Best Practices For Environmental Hygiene" by Linda Homan, Ecolab USA (2010), O.R. Environmental Hygiene, An Online Continuing Education Activity, sponsored by Pfiedler Enterprises, *www.pfiedlerenterprises.com* (2013), "The Power of Video Recording: Taking Quality to the Next Level," by Martin A. Makary

M.D., M.P.H. *Journal of The American Medical Association* (April 17, 2013) and see "An Electronic Eye on Hospital Hand-Washing," by Tina Rosenberg (November 24, 2011) detailing the experience in ICUs in North Shore University Hospital in Manhasset, New York. For the mortal and economic costs of infections see *Unnecessary Deaths: The Human and Financial Costs of Hospital Infections* by Betsy McCaughey, PhD (2006) which details the experiences in Pennsylvania hospitals, among others, and is published by RID, The Committee to Reduce Infection Deaths. Also see "Infection Control—A Problem for Patient Safety," by John P. Burke M.D., *New England Journal of Medicine* (February 13, 2003).

In terms of utilizing behavior modification tools to improve health care hygiene see "Culture Change and Infection Control: Applying Psychological Principles to Improve Hand Hygiene," by Ethan Cumbler, M.D., *Journal of Nursing Care Quality* (October/December 2013) vol. 28 issue 4. This paper details the experience in the Elderly Medicine Unit at the University of Colorado Hospital. For a favorable Hawaii experience see "Eradicating Central Line—associated Bloodstream Infections Statewide: The Hawaii Experience," by Della M. Lin M.D., MS., *American Journal of Medical Quality* (March/April 2012). An excellent resource for limiting and preventing infections is *Prevention of Hospital-Acquired Infections: A Practical Guide*, 2nd Edition, by the *World Health Organization, Department of Communicable Disease, Surveillance and Response* (2002). Also see "A Research Framework for Reducing Preventable Patient Harm," by Peter J. Pronovost et al. in *Clinical Infectious Diseases* (2011) 52 (4): 507–513, which delves into the Michigan and other initiatives to prevent central line–associated bloodstream infections (CLABSIs). Also see "An Intervention to Decrease Catheter Related Bloodstream Infections in the ICU," by Peter J. Pronovost et al. in *The New England Journal of Medicine* (December 28, 2006). *The Joint Commission International* has published "Preventing Central-Line Associated Bloodstream Infections, A Global Challenge, A Global Perspective" (2012). See "Q & A: Hospital Infection Rates Rarely Disclosed Despite Thousands of Deaths, More Killed Annually Than by Auto Accidents and Homicides," ABC News, October 14, 2005 and "Multi-State Point-Prevalent Survey of Health Care Associated Infections," by Shelly Magill, M.D., PhD et al. *New England Journal of Medicine* (March 27, 2014). For an analysis of MRSA contamination and how it was controlled see "Veteran's Affairs Initiative to Prevent Methicillin-Resistant *Staphylococcus aureus* Infections," by Rajiv Jain, M.D., et al., *New England Journal of Medicine* (April 14, 2011) and "Study Finds Drop In Deadly VA Hospital Infections," by Kevin Sack, *New York Times* (April 13, 2011). Also see "Perceived Strength of Evidence Supporting Practices to Prevent Healthcare-Associated Infection: Results From A National Survey of Infection Prevention Personnel," by Sanjay Saint M.D., M.P.H. et al. *American Journal of Infection Control* (February 2013) 41(2): 100–106, "Data Shows Scourge of Hospital Infections," by Ceci Connolly, *The Washington Post* (July 13, 2005), "Making Hospitals Pay for Their Mistakes," by Tara Parker-Pope, *The New York Times* (December 19, 2007), "Deadly Bacteria That Resists Strongest Drugs Are Spreading," by Denise Grady, *The New York Times* (March 5, 2013), "An Environmental Disinfection Odyssey: Evaluation of Sequential Interventions to Improve Disinfection of *Clostridium difficile* Isolation Rooms," by Brett Sitzlar et al., *Infection Control and Hospital Epidemiology* (May 20, 2013), "Deadly Bacteria That Defy Drugs of Last Resort," by Peter Eisler, *USA TODAY* (March 6, 2013). For surgical site infections see "Steps for Surgical Patients to Fight Infection," *the Wall Street Journal* (March 11, 2013). The Department of Health and Human Services also issued its "Action Plan to Prevent Healthcare-Associated Infections Including MRSA c. diff. Catheter Associated Urinary Tract Infections (CAUTI)," "Ventilator Associated Ammonias, Multi-Drug Resistant Organisms, etc." This is an important joint report dated June 2009 involving the Agency for Healthcare Research and Quality, the Office of the Assistant Secretary for Public Affairs, the Office of the Assistant Secretary for Planning and Evaluation, the Centers for Disease Control and Prevention, the Centers for Medicare & Medicaid Services, the Food and Drug Administration, the National Institutes of Health, the Office of the National Coordinator for Health Information Technology and the Office of Public Health and Science.

For M.P.H. United Kingdom's approach see, "Improving Patient Care by Reducing the Risk of Hospital Acquired Infection: A Progress Report," by the Comptroller and Auditor General, *National Audit Office* (July 14, 2004). The list of preventive measures that patients can apply that appear in this chapter are derived from the "World Health Organization Prevention Guide," "The Department of Health and Human Services Action Plan," suggestions that appear in his book *Safe Patients: Smart Hospitals* by Peter Pronovost, in a report by Betsy McCaughey PhD, "For The Committee to

Reduce Infection Deaths," and Robert Wachter's volume *Understanding Patient Safety.*

CHAPTER 11: BEDSORES AND BLOOD CLOTS

Regarding bedsores I learned much about the scope of the problem from a survey supplement in *The Annals of Internal Medicine* "Preventing In-Facility Pressure Ulcers As a Patient Safety Strategy, A Systematic Review," by Nancy Sullivan, BA and Karen M. Schoelles, M.D., SM (March 5, 2013). Information on the Braden Scale predicting pressure sore risk is published in the unified language system of the National Institutes of Health, see www.nlm.nih.gov. Also see "Predictive Validity of The Braden Scale Among Black and White Subjects," by N. Bergstrom, and B.J. Braden in *Nursing Research* (November/December 2002) and "Predictive Validity of The Braden Scale and Nurse Perception in Identifying Pressure Ulcer Risk," by T. VandenBosch et al., *Applied Nursing Research* (May 9, 1996). The Braden Scale has an official web site (www.bradenscale.com), an instruction sheet (www.healthcare.uiow.edu / igec/ tools/pressureulcers/bradenscale.pdf), and an assessment form (www.in.gov/isdh/files/braden_scale.pdf.) I learned about the scope of pressure ulcer and blood clot deaths from attending the "Best Practices and Patient-Centered Care Conference," at Johns Hopkins on September 26–27, 2013, in Baltimore, Maryland where nurses described tools and strategies for being alerted to turn and tend to patients. The Conference was a project of the Armstrong Institute for Patient Safety and Quality and supported by the United States Agency for Healthcare Research and Quality, and Betty Moore Foundation. Regarding the Medicare No Pay for Errors List, which includes stage III and IV pressure ulcers and certain types of blood clots, I learned about that as well as the medical issues pertaining to prevention of pulmonary emboli and deep vein thrombosis in *Understanding Patient Safety* by Robert M. Wachter, M.D., Pressure ulcer stages and position changing and cleaning were described in *The American College of Physicians Medical Knowledge Self-Assessment Program on General Internal Medicine* at pages 116–117. This book also introduced me to the pressure ulcer for healing (PUSH) scale and certain remedies including position changes, bedding that reduces pressure, and wound care, as well as certain still-experimental approaches like electrotherapy and hypobaric oxygen. Regarding embolism, this volume indicates that prophylactic measures prevent 50–80% of cases through the use of compression devices and certain anti-coagulants like low molecular weight heparin (LMWH). The vital involvement of the American College of Chest Physicians (ACCP) and it prophylactic strategies are also found in Robert Wachter *Understanding Patient Safety* at pages 180–181.

CHAPTER 12: DELIRIUM AND FALLS

For both delirium and falls I derived background from Wachter's *Understanding Patient Safety and The American College of Physicians Medical Knowledge Self-Assessment Program on General Internal Medicine*. *The Annals of Internal Medicine* had a helpful supplement analyzing multi-component delirium prevention programs entitled "In-Facility Delirium Prevention Programs as a Patient Safety Strategy: A Systematic Review," by James T. Reston, PhD, M.P.H. and Karen M. Schoelles, M.D., SM., found at Ann Intern Med. 2013; 158: 375–380. The Yale Hospitals Study is covered in "A Multicomponent Intervention to Prevent Delirium in Hospitalized Older Patients," by Sharon Inouye, M.D., M.P.H. et al. in the *New England Journal of Medicine* (March 4, 1999). For distinguishing delirium and dementia see "Delirium or Dementia?" by James L. Rudolph, M.D., SM, *Web M&M* (May 2009). For scoring delirium see "Clarifying Confusion: The Confusion Assessment Method. A New Method for Detection of Delirium," by Sharon K. Inouye, M.D., M.P.H. et al., *Annals of Internal Medicine* 1990; 113: 941–948. Also see "Delirium in The Intensive Care Unit: Occurrence and Clinical Course in Older Patients," by Lynn McNicoll, M.D., FRCPC in *The Journal of the American Geriatric Society* 51:591–598, 2003. For predicting delirium see "A Predictive Model for Delirium In Hospitalized Elderly Medical Patients Based on Admission Characteristics," by Sharon K. Inouye, M.D., M.P.H. et al. in *The Annals of Internal Medicine* (September 15, 1993), "Predicting Delirium in Elderly Patients: Development and Validation of a Risk-Stratification Model" by S.T. O'Keeffe and J.N. Lavan in *Age and Ageing* 1996; 25: 317–321. For outcome and prevention see "Does Delirium Contribute to Poor Hospital Outcomes? A Three-site Epidemiologic Study" by Sharon K. Inouye, M.D., M.P.H., et al. *Journal of General Internal Medicine* 1998 April; 13(4):234–42, and "Less is More, Potentially Inappropriate Medications Defined by STOPP Criteria and The Risk of Adverse Drug Events in Older Hospitalized Patients," by Hilary Hamilton, MB,MRCPI in *The Archives of Internal Medicine* (June 13, 2011). For delirium following trauma and surgery "Reducing Delirium After Hip Fracture: A Randomized Trial," by Edward. R. Marcantonio, M.D., SM, et al. in *The Journal of The American Geriatric Society* September 10, 2003 49:516–522.

On falls, "Will My Patient Fall?" by David A. Ganz, M.D., M.P.H. in the *Journal of The American Medical Association*, January 3, 2007; 297(1):77–86 was a seminal article for health care professionals. *The Annals of Internal Medicine* dedicated a supplement to falls: "Inpatient Fall Prevention Programs as a Patient Safety Strategy: A Systematic Review," by Isomi M. Miake-Lye, BA et al. (March 5, 2013). For evidence on falls increasing with age and length of hospital stay, "Fall Prevention in Acute Care Hospitals: A Randomized Trial," by Patricia C. Dykes, RN, DNSC, et al. in *Journal of the American Medical Association* (November 3, 2010). Regarding the hip protector controversy see "Efficacy of a Hip-Protector to Prevent Hip Fracture in Nursing Home Residents: The HIP PRO Randomized Controlled Trial," by Douglas P. Kiel, M.D., M.P.H. et al. in the *Journal of The American Medical Association* (July 25, 2007) and "Expression of Concern: Kiel et al. Efficacy of a Hip-Protector to Prevent Hip Fracture in Nursing Home Residents: The HIP PRO Randomized Controlled Trial," by Howard Bauchner, M.D., and Phillip B. Fontanarosa, M.D., MBA, *Journal of The American Medical Association* 2007; 298(4): 413–422.

The STRATIFY risk assessment tool and its use were included by Robert M. Wachter in *Understanding Patient Safety* pages 182–183.

CHAPTER 13: THE HEALTH-CARE ENVIRONMENT SHOULD BE CLEAN AND RATIONAL

For more on Earle H. Spaulding see "Principles and Application of Chemical Disinfection" by Spaulding in *The Journal of the Association of Operating Room Nurses* (AORN) (May/June 1963) and "Alcohol As a Surgical Disinfectant," *Journal of the Association of Operating Room Nurses* (AORN) (September/October 1964). The obituary of "Earle H. Spaulding, 88, Microbiologist" by Andy Wallace appeared in the *Philadelphia Inquirer* on February 4, 1995. Information regarding CDC standards principally comes from "Guidelines For Environmental Infection Control in Healthcare Facilities" (Recommendations of CDC and the Healthcare Infection Control Practices Advisory Committee) (HICPAC) by The U.S. Department of Health and Human Services Centers for Disease Control and Prevention (CDC) Atlanta, Georgia (2003). Also see "2007 Guideline For Isolation Precautions: Preventing Transmission of Infectious Agents in Healthcare Settings," by Jane D. Siegel, M.D., et al. Also see "Management of Multi-Drug Resistant Organisms in Healthcare Settings, 2006 by Jane D. Siegel, M.D., published by the Centers for Disease Control and Prevention and "Guideline for Infection Control in Healthcare Personnel," (1998) by Elizabeth A. Bolyard, RN, M.P.H., Centers for Disease Control and Prevention. Also see "Guideline For Disinfection and Sterilization in Healthcare Facilities," Centers for Disease Control and Prevention, 2008, which notes Earle H. Spaulding's contribution and also articulates methods for dealing with critical items, semi-critical items, and non-critical items. This CDC Guideline reflects changes in disinfection and sterilization since 1981. The CDC published "Options for Evaluating Environmental Cleaning," prepared by Alice Guh, M.D., M.P.H. and Phillip Carling, M.D., in December 2010. For automation of cleaning see "Infection Rates Drop at West Chester Medical Center When Pulsed Xenon UV Used to Disinfect Rooms; 3rd Xenox Customer Reports HAI Reduction in Peer-Reviewed Literature," Business Wire June 2, 2014, "The Role of 'No-Touch' Automated Room Disinfection Systems in Infection Prevention and Control," by J. A. Otter et al., *Journal of Hospital Infection* 2013 Jan; 83(1): 1–13, "UV Robots Zap Germs and Disinfect Rooms at UPMC Hospitals," a press release distributed on rounds at UPMC July 9, 2014, "Violet The Robot Attacks Germs At UPMC Passavant," by Yanan Wang, *Pittsburgh Post-Gazette* (July 9, 2014), "Hospitals Turn to Cleaning 'Robots' to Fight Superbugs," *Associated Press*, April 29, 2013, which is an article that surveys the experience with these machines in a host of settings and hospitals including Westchester Medical Center and Lenox Hill Hospital in New York, "Role of Ultra-Violet (UV) Disinfection in Infection Control and Environmental Cleaning," by Z. Qureshi, and M.H. Yassin, in *Infectious Disorder Drug Targets* (June 2013), "Implementation and Impact of Ultraviolet Environmental Disinfection in an Acute Care Setting," by Janet P. Haas, PhD, RN, et al., *American Journal of Infection Control* 42 (2014)586–90, "Western PA Hospitals Test Robot Using Ultraviolet Rays to Kill Bacteria," by Adam Smeltz, *Pittsburgh Tribune Review* (July 9, 2014). On the effect of surfaces see "The Role of Surface Environment in Healthcare-Associated Infections," by David J. Weber, Deverick Anderson and William A. Rutala, in *Current Opinion in Infectious Disease* 2013; 26(4): 338–344.

For the role of the United States Occupational Safety and Health Administration (OSHA) see "Blood Borne Pathogens Standard and Disinfection," by Tom Bach in *Infection Control Today* (September 1, 2000). The CDC has an extensive infection control glossary that I found useful. It can be found at www.cdc.gov/oralhealth/infectioncontrol/glossary.htm.

General articles on modern hospital cleaning methods include "Hospital Cleaning in the 21st Century," by S. J. Dancer in *The European Journal of Microbiology and Infectious Diseases* (April 17, 2011), "Cleaning the Hospital Environment—A Focus on Difficle-S," by Maurice Madeo, in *The British Journal of Nursing* (2011) Vol. 20, no. 11, and "A Microbiological Evaluation of Hospital Cleaning Methods," by Liza F. White, et al., *International Journal of Environmental Health Research*, 2007 August; 17(4): 285–95.

Regarding design of hospital facilities see especially "Fable Hospital 2.0: The Business Case for Building Better Hospital Facilities," by Blair H. Saddler et al. in *Hastings Center Report* (January/February 2011), "The Application of Hospitality Elements in Hospitals," by Ziqi Wu, *Journal of Healthcare Management* 58: 1, January/February 2013, "How to Help Hospitals Achieve Their Mission Through Good Design," by Barry S. Rabner, M.P.H.A *Health Environments Research & Design Journal* Vol. 5, no. 3, Spring 2012. This is an interesting piece on how the 220-bed acute-care hospital in Princeton was strategically rebuilt according to rational care principles. Also see "Patients and Their Families Weigh In On Evidence-Based Hospital Design," by Kathleen Trochelman, RN, MSN in *Critical Care Nurse* (February 2012) and "Acuity-Adaptable Nursing Care: Exploring Its Place in Designing the Future Patient Room," by Melissa A. Kwan, M.P.H., *Health Environments Research and Design Journal* Vol. 5 no. 1, Fall 2011. For the effects of design on health-care personnel see "Environmental Congruence and Work-Related Stress in Acute Care Hospitals Medical/Surgical Units: A Descriptive, Correlational Study," by Nancy Dendaas, RN, PhD in *Health Environments Research and Design Journal* Vol. 5 No. 1, Fall 2011.

CHAPTER 14: HEALTH-CARE ENVIRONMENT SHOULD BE OPEN AND OVERSEEN

Florence Nightingale was referenced in *The Greatest Benefit to Mankind*, by Roy Porter, W.W. Norton (1999). Ernest Amory Codman came up in *Unaccountable*, by Marty Makary, M.D., Bloomsbury Press (2012). The contributions of both figures to the issue of reporting error also arose in the coronary artery bypass graft literature which placed them as reporters in context. See in particular "Public Reporting of Cardiac Surgery Performance: Part 1—History, Rationale, Consequences," by David M. Shahian, M.D., et al., in the *Annals of Thoracic Surgery*, 2011; 92 S2–S11. The CABG reporting reforms have been written about extensively; see "The Decline in Coronary Artery Bypass Graft Surgery Mortality in New York State, The Role of Surgeon Volume," by Edward L. Hannan, PhD, et al. *Journal of The American Medical Association* (January 18, 1995), "Report on Coronary Artery Bypass Surgery Shows Consistent Quality Care Throughout New York State, Overall Risk-Adjusted Mortality Rates CABG Remain Low," by *The New York State Health Department* (November 7, 2002), "The Predictive Accuracy of The New York State Coronary Artery Bypass Surgery Report-Card System, What Impact Has The New York State CABG Reporting System Had on Market Share and Surgical Practice?" by Ashish K. Jha and Arnold M. Epstein in *HealthAffairs* Vol. 25 No.3 (May/June 2006), "The Impact of Mandatory Public Reporting on Coronary Artery Bypass Graft (CABG) Case Selection and Outcomes in California," by The University of California, Davis Study Consultant Team, Patrick Romano, M.D., M.P.H., et al. (February 2010), "The New York State Cardiac Registries: History, Contributions, Limitations, and Lessons for Future Efforts to Assess and Publicly Report Healthcare Outcomes," by Edward L. Hannan, PhD et al., *Journal of The American College of Cardiology* Vol. 59 No. 25, 2012. Also see "Public Reporting of Cardiac Surgery Performance: Part II—Implementation," by David M. Shahian, M.D., et al., in the Annals of Thoracic Surgery, 2011; 92: S12–S23, and "New York State's Cardiac Surgery Reporting System: Four Years Later," by Edward L. Hannan, PhD *et al., Annals of Thoracic Surgery* 1994; 58: 1852–7. For an excellent brief recent memoir of CABG surgery, see "A Broken Chest Is Better Than a Broken Heart" by Sed Kurtz, *Pittsburgh Post-Gazette* (January 17, 2015).

The National Healthcare Quality Report is published annually by the *Agency For Healthcare Research and Quality of The U.S. Department of Health and Human Services*, the May 2014 Report is AHRQ No. 14–0005 and is found at www.ahrq.gov/research/findings/nhqrdr/index.html. *The Office of the Inspector General in the Department of Health and Human Services* has issued two important reports: "Adverse Events in Hospitals: Case Study of Incidence Among Medicare Beneficiaries in Two Selected Counties," by Daniel R. Levinson, Inspector General (December 2008), and "Hospital Incident Reporting Systems Do Not Capture Most Patient Harm," by Daniel R. Levinson, Inspector General (January 2012). Also see a significant follow-up memorandum "Few Adverse Events in Hospitals Were Reported to State Adverse Event Reporting Systems," Stuart Wright, Deputy Inspector General for Evaluation and Inspections, to Marilyn Tavenner, Acting Administrator Centers for Medicare and Medicaid Services (July 19, 2012). This is the document that points out the high level of reporting, indeed that of half the reporting of incidents by all hospitals to state agencies occurs in just one state, Pennsylvania. For the Pennsylvania experience, see the "Pennsylvania Patient Safety Authority 2013 Annual Report," dated April 30, 2014 submitted by Carrie DeLone, M.D., Physician General and Chair, Board of Directors Pennsylvania Patient Safety Authority. For a website detailing all 50 States' Reporting Practices or lack thereof, see QUPS.org.

For the Joint Commission National Patient Safety Goals for Hospitals plus other standards go to http://www.jointcommission.org. Regarding the Accreditation Council for Graduate Medical Education (ACGME) I reviewed the ACGME Common Program Requirements effective July 1, 2013. In *Understanding Patient Safety*, Robert M. Wachter M.D., wrote about Patient Safety Organizations (PSOs) and the Patient Safety and Quality Improvement Act of 2005. The issue also came up in the 2013 National Healthcare Quality Report by The Agency for Healthcare Research and Quality. A reform-oriented hospital leader, T. Michael White, M.D., shared his positive views about PSOs in discussions with me in November and December 2014. For Medicare Bounce-backs see "Hospitals Here, Nationwide Penalized for Patient Readmissions," by Henry Davis, *The Buffalo News* (January 31, 2013), "Hospitals Face Pressure to Avert Readmissions," by Jordan Rau, *The New York Times* (November 26, 2012), "Medicare's Decision to Withhold Payment for Hospital Errors: The Devil Is in the Details," by Robert M. Wachter, M.D., Nancy E. Foster, and R. Adams Dudley, M.D., MBA *The Joint Commission Journal on Quality and Patient Safety*, Vol. 34, No. 2 February 2008, pp. 116–123, "Non-Payment for Harms Resulting From Medical Care Catheter-Associated Urinary Tract Infections," by Heidi L. Wald, M.D., MSPH, and Andrew M. Cramer, M.D., *Journal of The American Medical Association* (December 19, 2007).

Pertaining to malpractice see "Relation Between Malpractice Claims and Adverse Events Due to Negligence: Results of the Harvard Medical

Practice Study III," by A. Russell Localio, JD, M.P.H., et al. *New England Journal of Medicine* (July 25, 1991), *Medical Negligence: The Role of America's Civil Justice System in Protecting Patients' Rights*, American Association for Justice (February 2011), "Doctors Appeal Rulings That Diminish Error Reporting Protections," by Alicia Gallegos, November 19, 2012 in *American Medical News. Respectful Management of Serious Clinical Adverse Events, Innovation Series 2010*, by The Institute for Healthcare Improvement.

The writing on tort reform is voluminous. Some articles that state various positions in detailed ways include "Evaluating The Medical Malpractice System and Options for Reform," by Daniel P. Kessler *The Journal of Economic Perspective* (October 17, 2011), "Let's Make a Deal: Trading Malpractice Reform for Health Reform," by William M. Sage and David A. Hyman, *HealthAffairs* (January 2014), "Medical Malpractice Tort Reform," by David M. Ottenwes, Esquire et al., in *Radiology Management* (March/April 2011), "In Medical Malpractice and Tort Reform: Yes, Deal Better With the Issues But Don't Get Sidelined For More Costly, Needed Healthcare Reforms," by Glenn D. Braunstein, M.D., *Huffington Post* (August 13, 2012). For an analysis of tort reform by The Congressional Budget Office see a letter to Senator Orrin G. Hatch from Douglas W. Elmendorf, Director Congressional Budget Office, August 9, 2009.

The seminal article both in terms of tort reform but also using malpractice to estimate overall medical errors, which became instrumental in the Harvard Medical Malpractice Study, The British Medical Study and other analyses of the National Practitioners Data Bank is "Medical Insurance Feasibility Study: A Technical Summary," by Don Harper Mills M.D., JD in *The Western Journal of Medicine* (April 1978).

For Health Courts and other alternative Tribunals, see "Patient Safety, Risk Reduction, and the Law," by Larry I. Palmer, 36 Huston Law Review 1609(1999), "Health Courts and Accountability for Patient Safety," by Michelle M. Mello et al., *The Milbank Quarterly*, Vol. 84, No. 3, 2006, "Why Health Courts are Unconstitutional," by Amy Widman *27 Pace Law Review 55* (2006), "Give Health Courts a Fair Shake," by Mark Crane, *The Journal of The American Enterprise Institute* (August 20, 2007), and "Administrative Compensation for Medical Injuries: Lessons from Three Foreign Systems," by Michelle M. Mello et al., *The Commonwealth Fund* 1517 Vol. 14 (July 2001). I discussed the "dizzy" stroke trial with malpractice attorney Alan Perer on various occasions during December 2014 and January 2015. A particularly good survey article on health courts and other non-trial options is "Administrative Compensation of Medical Injuries: A Hardy Perennial Blooms Again," by Paul Barringer, et al. *Journal of Health Politics Policy and Law* (August 2008). The reference to $50 million dollars set aside for States to explore Health Courts was reported in "Let's Make a Deal: Trading Malpractice Reform for Health Reform," by William M. Sage and David A. Hyman, *HealthAffairs* (January 2014).

Writing pertaining to efforts to stop over practice and over treatment leading to injuries includes "Medical Malpractice: Why is it so Hard for Doctors to Apologize? Fixing a System Built on Blame and Revenge Will Require Bold Ways of Analyzing Mistakes and a Radical Embrace of Openness," by Dr. Darshak Sanghavi, *The Boston Globe* (January 27, 2013), "Defensive Medicine Among High-Risk Specialist Physicians in a Volatile Malpractice Environment," by David M. Studdert, LLB,ScD, M.P.H. et al. *Journal of The American Medical Association* (June 1, 2005), "To Improve US Health Care, Heed MD-Specialists' Suggestions to Reduce Excess Tests," by Glenn D. Braunstein, M.D., *Huffington Post* (April 9, 2012), "More Treatment, More Mistakes," by Sanjay Gupta, *The New York Times* (July 31, 2012).

Regarding the popularity of Centers for Medicare and Medicaid Services (CMS) see "Americans Like Medicare and Medicaid but Parties Split on Expansion," by Kathy Frankovic, *Economist/YOUGOV Poll* (September 8, 2014). Chesley B. Sullenberger, II gave his speech "Islands of Excellence in a Sea of System Failure: Why Healthcare Needs to Adapt Lessons From Aviation," at Johns Hopkins on September 13, 2013.

The I-Pass System was studied and described in "Changes in Medical Errors after Implementation of a Handoff Program," by Amy J. Starmer, M.D., M.P.H., et al., *New England Journal of Medicine* (November 6, 2014).

For the Indianapolis Colonoscopy Surveillance Study see "The Impact of Video Recording on the Quality of Colonoscopy Performance, A Pilot Study," by Douglas K. Rex, M.D., *The American Journal of Gastroenterology* (November 2010) and "Patient Interest in Video Recording of Colonoscopy: A Survey," by Meghana Raghavendra, and Douglas K. Rex, *World Journal of Gastroenterology* (August 18, 2009).

Root cause analysis is described in *Unsafe to Safe: An Impatient Proposal for Safe Patient-Centered Care* by T. Michael White M.D., 2012 and in *Understanding Patient Safety* by Robert M. Wachter. I discussed root cause analysis with T. Michael White M.D., during January and February 2015.

The Patient Safety Indicators (PSIs) are produced by the Agency for Healthcare Research and Quality. The National Quality Forum is a private/public partnership non-profit organization including individuals and health-care business and government. Its standards are highly respected and grew out of its earlier list of so-called "never events."

T. Michael White also discussed with me his use of personal/professional patient advocates (P3As) during interviews in January 2015. Issues of nursing ratios, reporting accidents as is done in other industries, and communications between health-care professionals and patients including Teaching Back and empathy arose at the Best Practices in Patient Centered Care Conference September 26–27, 2013 at Baltimore Maryland, sponsored by the Armstrong Institute for Patient Safety and Quality at Johns Hopkins where Peter J. Pronovost gave the Keynote Speech on "Safety Quality and Patient-Centered Care."

Selected Bibliography

Aboumatar, Hanan, J., M.D., and Peter J. Pronovost, M.D. (2013, September). *Best Practices in Patient-Centered Care Conference*. Conducted at the Armstrong Institute for Patient Safety and Quality, Baltimore, M.D.

Ackerknecht, Derwin H. M.D., *A Short History of Medicine*, Rev. ed. Baltimore, M.D.: Johns Hopkins University Press, 1982

Adams, Karen and Janet M. Corrigan, Eds. *Priority Areas for National Action: Transforming Care Quality*. Washington, DC: National Academies Press, 2003

Accreditation Council for Graduate Medical Education. *Common Program Requirements*. Chicago, IL: 2013

American College of Physicians. *MKSAP 14: Medical Knowledge Self-Assessment Program Part A*. Philadelphia, PA: American College of Physicians, 2006

American College of Physicians. *MKSAP 14: Medical Knowledge Self-Assessment Program Part B*. Philadelphia, PA: American College of Physicians, 2006

Aspden, Philip, et al. *Patient Safety: Achieving a New Standard for Care*. Washington, DC: National Academies Press, 2004

Aspden, Philip, et al. *Preventing Medication Errors: Quality Chasm Series*. Washington, DC: National Academies Press, 2007

Bennett, Claude J., M.D., and Fred Plum, M.D., et al. *Cecil Textbook of Medicine, 20th Ed. Vol. 1*. Philadelphia, PA: Harcourt Brace, 1996

Bennett, Claude J., M.D., and Fred Plum, M.D., et al. *Cecil Textbook of Medicine, 20th Ed. Vol. 2*. Philadelphia, PA: Harcourt Brace, 1996

Boyland, Elizabeth A., RN, et al. "Guideline for Infection Control in Health Care Personnel, 1998." *American Journal of Infection Control 26, no. 3 (1998)*: 289–354

Brunwald, Eugene, M.D., et al. *Harrison's Manual of Medicine*, 15th Ed. New York: McGraw-Hill, 2002

Brawley, Otis Webb, M.D., with Paul Goldberg. *How We Do Harm: A Doctor Breaks Ranks About Being Sick in America.* New York: St. Martin's Griffin, 2012

Brownlie, Shannon. *Overtreated: Why Too Much Medicine Is Making Us Sicker and Poorer.* New York: Bloomsbury USA, 2007

Bynum, William. *The History of Medicine: A Very Short Introduction*. New York: Oxford University Press, 2008

CDC and HealthCare Infection Control Practices Advisory Committee. *Guidelines for Environmental Infection Control in Health-Care Facilities*. Atlanta, GA: Centers for Disease Control, 2003

Centers for Disease Control and Prevention. "Trends in Tuberculosis—United States, 2008" *MMWR 58, no. 10 (2009):* 249–276

Charney, William, Ed. *Epidemic of Medical Errors and Hospital-Acquired Infections Systemic and Social Causes.* Boca Raton, FL: CRC Press

Committee on Quality of Health Care In America. *Crossing the Quality Chasm: A New Health System for the 21st Century.* Washington, DC: National Academy Press 1998

Committees on Redesigning Health Insurance Performance Measures, Payment and Performance. *Rewarding Provider Performance: Aligning Incentives in Medicare.* Washington, DC: National Academies Press, 2007

Corrigan, Janet M, Ann Greiner, and Shari M. Erickson, Eds. *Fostering Rapid Advances in Health Care: Learning From System Demonstrations.* Washington, DC: National Academies Press, 2013

Ferri, Fred F., M.D., *Practical Guide to the Care of the Medical Patient, 3rd Ed*. St. Louis, MO: Mosby-Year Book, Inc., 1991

Gawande, Atul. *The Checklist Manifesto: How To Get Things Right*. New York: Henry Holt & Co., 2009

Gawande, Atul. *Complications: A Surgeon's Notes On An Imperfect Science*. New York: Henry Holt & Co., 2002

Hosh, Amit K., M.D., Ed. *Mayo Clinic Internal Medicine Review, 8th Ed*. Rochester, MN: Scientific Publications

Graban, Mark. *Lean Hospitals: Improving Quality, Patient Safety and Employee Engagement, 2nd Ed*. Boca Raton, FL: CRC Press, 2012

Green, Gopa, M.D., et al., Ed. *The Washington Manual of Medical Therapeutics, 31st Ed*., Philadelphia, PA: Lippincott, Williams & Wilkins, 2002

Healthcare Infection Control Practices Advisory Committee. *Guidelines for Environmental Infection Control in Health-Care Facilities.* Atlanta, GA: Centers for Disease Control, 2003

Hurford, Williams, et al., Ed. *Critical Care Handbook of the Massachusetts General Hospital*. Philadelphia, PA: Lippincott, Williams & Wilkins, 2000

Iverson, Leslie. *Drugs: A Very Short Introduction*. New York: Oxford University Press, 2001

Kenney, Charles. *Transforming Health Care: Virginia Mason Medical Center's Pursuit of the Perfect Patient Experience*. Boca Raton, FL: CRC Press

King, Sorrel. *Josie's Story: A Mother's Inspiring Crusade to Make Medical Care Safe*. New York: Grove Press, 2009

Kohn, Linda T. et al., Ed. *To Err Is Human: Building a Smart Health System*. Washington, DC: National Academy Press, 2000

Makary, Marty, M.D., *Unaccountable: What Hospitals Won't Tell You and How Transparency Can Revolutionize Health Care*. New York: Bloomsbury Press, 2012

Mangram, Alicia J., M.D., et al. "Guideline for Prevention of Surgical Site Infection, 1999." *Infection Control and Hospital Epidemiology* 20, no. 4 (1999): 247–278

McKibben, Linda, M.D., et al. Guidance on Public Reporting of Healthcare-Associated Infections: "Recommendations of the Healthcare Infection Control Practices Advisory Committee." *American Journal of Infection Control 33, no. 4* (2005): 217–226

Millenson, Michael. *Demanding Medical Excellence: Doctors and Accountability in the Information Age*. Chicago, IL: University of Chicago Press, 1997

Nader, Ralph. *Unsafe at Any Speed: The Designed-In Dangers of the American Automobile*. New York, Simon and Schuster, 1965

Page, Ann, Ed. Keeping Patients Safe: Transforming the Work Environment of Nurses. Washington, DC: National Academies Press, 2004

PDR Staff. *The PDR Pocket Guide to Prescription Drugs, 10th Ed*. Montvale, NJ: PDR Network.

Porter, Roy, Ed. *Cambridge Illustrated History of Medicine*. New York: Cambridge University Press, 1998

Porter, Roy. *The Greatest Benefit to Mankind: A Medical History of Humanity*. New York: W. W. Norton, 1999

Pronovost, Peter, M.D., and Eric Vohr. *Safe Patient, Smart Hospitals: How One Doctor's Checklist Can Help Us Change Healthcare From the Inside Out*. New York: Plume Books, 2011

Rutala, William A., Ph.D., et al. *Guideline for Disinfection and Sterilizations in Healthcare Facilities, 2008*. Atlanta, GA: Center for Disease Control, 2008

Schneider, Mary Jane. *Introduction to Public Health, 3rd Ed*. Sudbury, MA: Jones & Bartlett Publishing, 2011

Siegel, Jane D., M.D., et al. *2007 Guideline for Isolation Precautions: Preventing Transmission of Infectious Agents in Healthcare Settings*. Atlanta, GA: Center for Disease Control, 2007

Siegel, Jane D., M.D., et al. *Management of Multidrug-Resistant Organisms In Healthcare Settings, 2006*. Atlanta, GA: Center for Disease Control, 2006

Smith, Mark, et al., Ed. *Best Care at Lower Cost: The Path to Continuously Learning Health Care in America*. Washington, DC: National Academies Press, 2012

Thomas, Clayton, L., M.D., Ed. *Taber's Cyclopedic Medical Dictionary, 14th Ed*. Philadelphia, PA: F. A. Davis, 1981

Wachter, Robert M., M.D., *Understanding Patient Safety, 2nd Ed*. New York: McGraw-Hill, 2012

Williams, William, J. *Williams' Hematology Companion Handbook, 5th Ed*. New York: McGraw-Hill, 1995

Acknowledgments

Many people helped make this book possible by providing me with insights, information, and research. I would particularly like to thank Barbara Brown, Stacie Byers, D.O., Michael Diamond, M.D., Jodi Gill, Maribeth Hamel, Malcom Harris, M.D., Ruth Hart, John Kimmel, Anne Lieber, Paul Lieber, M.D., Barbara Mittleman, M.D., Maria Magone, Ph.D., Melvin Moten, Kristien Stevens, N.P., David E. Newman-Toker, M.D., Ph.D., Peter Pronovost, M.D., Ph.D., Louise Su, Bruce Wasser, T. Michael White, M.D., Jane Witt, and Carol Zisowitz, M.D., Ph.D.

My daughter Sara Green, herself an editor and writer, supplied the title. My wife, Margie Hammer, provided endless encouragement and support.

My editor John Oakes furnished able judgment and personified the courage of an independent publisher.

Index

Index (Organizations)

Index (People)

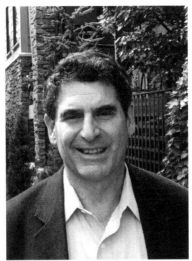

Author photograph by Ruth Hurt

ABOUT THE AUTHOR

James B. Lieber is the author of *Rats in the Grain: The Dirty Tricks and Trials of Archer Daniels Midland* and *Friendly Takeover: How an Employee Buyout Saved a Steel Town* (nominated for the Pulitzer Prize). He has written for a variety of publications, *The New York Times*, *The Atlantic Monthly*, and *The Nation* among them. His article on the financial crisis for *The Village Voice* became that publication's most widely read article for the year. He is a Pittsburgh-based lawyer, dividing his practice between civil rights law and commercial litigation.